FORGOTTEN FACES

Family Caregiver Voices

ROBERT W. TILLER

ISBN 978-1-64471-997-8 (Paperback)
ISBN 978-1-64471-998-5 (Hardcover)
ISBN 978-1-64471-999-2 (Digital)

Cover images used by permission and provided by:
©Can Stock Photo

Covenant Books, Inc.
11661 Hwy 707
Murrells Inlet, SC 29576
www.covenantbooks.com

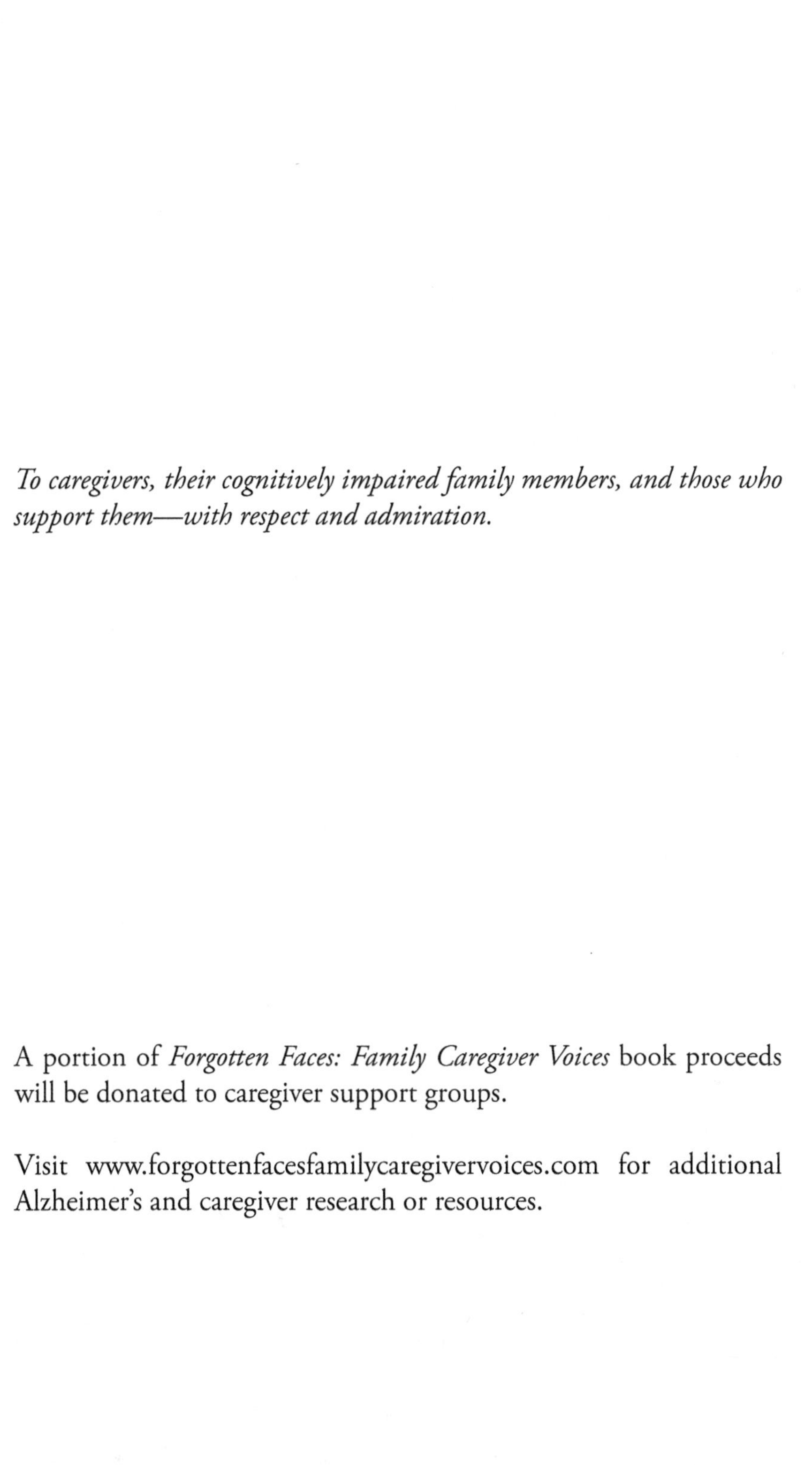

To caregivers, their cognitively impaired family members, and those who support them—with respect and admiration.

Forgotten Faces: Family Caregiver Voices

"It's personal. It's insightful. It's informative. And it could easily break your heart. Be prepared to be drawn into a world where many have been and many are going."
—RICHARD WILL, PhD

CONTENTS

FOREWORD

Forgotten Faces: Family Caregiver Voices explores the actual experiences of current and former caregivers to cognitively impaired family members. These stories reflect the blended voices of 24 actual caregivers. The caregivers and four industry professionals were individually interviewed as part of a research study conducted by a major university on the West Coast of Florida in 2017.[1] The events, emotions, and comments presented are the author's firsthand observations and the participants' actual quotations, with only names, tense, or gender modifications to protect their true identities.[2]

The caregivers' stories are presented first so readers may identify with their experiences, then learn why understanding their circumstances is so vital, followed by a behind-the-scenes look at the research science utilized to assure the book's trustworthiness.[3]

Although *Forgotten Faces* is a research-informed book, it was written in a nonacademic voice to inform multiple audiences in a more engaging manner.[4]

The text was formatted to avoid disruptive research notations and participant identifier references from interfering with readers' progress through the book. Instead, numbers placed inside the text correspond to such items within a *Notes* section. The *Notes* section includes additional author's commentary, broader explanations, scientific definitions, pertinent research items and references—sequentially presented to numerically correspond with their appearance throughout the text.

Forgotten Faces was researched and written by a practitioner scholar,[5] as part of a doctoral dissertation project,[6] intended to enhance and leverage his Alzheimer's and dementia caregiver subject knowledge from three decades of personal finance industry experience working with individual families.[7]

The caregiver study and book project were a prescriptive research effort[8] to:

- Create awareness of an enormous challenge awaiting our nation
- Evoke empathy for those who experience it
- Advocate action by families and policymakers to prepare while other researchers continue their valiant efforts to combat the disease

Love Thy Stranger

Friendly Faces

"Princess, get down!" ordered the tall, tanned, gray-haired man. He was embarrassed when his cat leaped onto the kitchen table and stepped on my notepad while I was setting up the audio recorder.

"Sorry about that," Fred said with a forced smile, "she just doesn't get to see many people." Princess returned to the floor, where she rubbed against the suit jacket I had hung on the back of my chair after realizing the home's windows were open to capture any warm, Florida East Coast cross-breezes.

As Fred politely offered me an iced tea, my eyes carefully canvased the dark, quiet house, and I sensed the cat was not the only one lonely for Mary, his wife of 56 years.

* * *

On Florida's West Coast, Janice nervously eyed the table's box of tissues so prominently lit by the fluorescent lighting of the public library's small conference room.

"I don't know where to begin," she said, before I even had the chance to ask when she first noticed her recently passed second husband was having some cognitive problems.

I could see Janice was eager to tell me about George—her magnificent midlife romance, her greatest hero and biggest heartache.

* * *

Alice looked past me, through her office's closed glass door, seemingly assessing the likelihood we would be spared interruptions from her bustling staff during our meeting.

"I know your schedule is tight," I said to Alice, "but this is your session—and I assure you whatever time you can spend with me today is appreciated." I moved my watch from wrist to the table—so I could monitor our session's length but view her nonverbal cues and read her emotions through frequent eye contact.[9]

As I filed her consent form alongside the others, I thanked Alice for volunteering to talk about taking care of her mother, Audrey, in my research study on caregivers to a cognitively impaired family member.[10]

* * *

"Oops, sorry," said Yvonne when she flopped her extra-large purse onto the library's community room table. "I only had time to grab these." Then she hurriedly set up an impromptu life history of her grandfather, Richard, with several loose photos and a couple of large portrait frames.

She smiled proudly and said if we were going to talk about her taking care of her grandfather—it was important to her that I see him for myself.

When I thanked her for bringing the photos, Yvonne said she forgot to bring her grandfather's brain scan[11]—and offered to send it if it would help with my research study.

Researcher's Note

As an unknown researcher to these volunteer case study participants, I found myself pleased, humbled, and honored they so willingly offered to discuss their heartfelt experiences of caring for their loved ones. I hoped the information these caregivers would share might provide a new perspective for those who have not yet experienced the phenomenon[12] of caring for a cognitively impaired family member.

I knew my data needed to be gathered and reported in an unbiased manner to be considered scientific research.[13] Yet I believed my decades of guiding families dealing with Alzheimer's or dementia, and having multiple incidents within my own family, would strengthen my ability to understand these participants.[14] To keep from influencing their responses, I deferred sharing my personal connection to this prescriptive research effort until after we had concluded their interviews.

With no promise other than an earnest effort to share their journey with whoever might read an intended book[15]—each of them seemed genuinely grateful to find someone interested in hearing their family's story.

Before the Storm

Fred sat down at the kitchen table, with Princess settled at his feet, ready to talk openly about his experience as Mary's caregiver. Fred was by no means a frail retiree, but he did appear physically and emotionally worn down—like a man toiling away at a task with no end in sight, but fully committed to its pursuit regardless. He spoke lovingly about his wife and family. Even as Fred described the past five years of dealing with the mounting challenges of Mary's Alzheimer's disease—his words were bittersweet but without bitterness. Fred managed to care for her at home the first three years, but Mary was already in a local memory ward for two years before our meeting.

He first told me of their happy retirement decision to reward themselves by moving south. They had packed up what they could, sold off what they could not, and drove down to spend their golden years enjoying the warm Florida weather and each other's company. He smiled back when I offered him a belated welcome to the state and told him I was a native Floridian myself, but I had "imported my wife from Long Island!"

When I asked him to recall some odd instances with Mary's cognition prior to her diagnosis, Fred said, "I saw a number of things happening that were troubling for me. I couldn't put a name on it but it just started to accumulate."[16]

He described his wife as a "voracious reader." Then, one night they were in bed reading, and he was perplexed to see Mary "was taking notes." He asked, "What are you doing?" He said her response was, "Well, I can't always remember what happened in the preceding pages, so…" Upon hindsight, Fred said that "was one little indication" that something was wrong.[17]

Around that same time, Fred recalled that although they often drove across several states to visit their daughter—once there, Mary would no longer take the car to run errands on her own. "Suddenly one year she said, 'Go with me.' So, I just thought she forgot how to do it. It's been more than a year, but that was the first time of not wanting to drive, not being able to drive, but not saying that. She just said, 'Would you go with me?' So, I took her there, came back. It's one of these things I've learned after the fact that, you get these signs but you don't understand it, you don't react to it."[18]

Fred's eyes looked to mine for affirmation that it may have seemed reasonable not to have recognized Mary's early behaviors as forecasting significant problems ahead. In keeping with established research interviewing methods,[19] I kept my gaze focused upon him to see the emotion of *how* he was speaking—secure in the knowledge that the audio recorder would provide an accurate transcription of *what* he was saying.

Mary's memory issues continued beyond Fred's earlier dismissals. He noticed she stopped cooking and complained about the kitchen—saying, "The stuff isn't organized, it's too far away." In hindsight, he said it was that Mary "couldn't remember by the time she went across the room to get—whether she was supposed to get a pan, or (something else)."[20]

Eventually others helped Fred recognize that something was wrong. "She would lose her billfold or her purse…just unusually poor memory for a person who was bright…started losing things and forgetting what I told her. I thought, 'Well maybe I'm overreacting.' We had some very good friends—we went on a week vacation to the beach together, which was normally what we did. I said, 'You know I'm concerned about Mary.' These are people who have known her our whole lives. They, after the week, they said, 'Yeah, we noticed some things.'"[21]

Tears welled in Fred's eyes as he revealed the moment he finally realized he could not deny Mary's problem any longer. He said, "The biggest thing was…we had our 50th wedding anniversary and I literally begged her, 'Let's do something special! Let's go to Charleston, South Carolina, or New Orleans or someplace like that.' She didn't want to go, she didn't want to go. Couldn't get her to go. We ended up having dinner at the Red Lobster. And then a week later, she was talking to my daughter and said, 'We had our 50th anniversary—we should have done something! Why didn't we do something special or something?' So then I knew that, that was the big thing…'Okay, we got a real problem here.'"[22]

Things grew worse as Fred realized the potential dangers of ignoring Mary's undiagnosed cognitive problem when he asked her about the checkbook. "I said, 'How much money do we have?' She said, 'I don't know…I don't know how much money we've got.' I said, 'What do you mean you don't know how much money we've got?' (Mary said), 'Well, I took the check register to the bank and they've got it.' I said, 'What! How long have they had it?' She says, 'Well, I don't know. Maybe two weeks.' And I said, 'Well…we've got to go to the bank.' Sure enough, they had it. I said, 'Well, how much money did we have?' (The bank employee said), 'That question I can answer. You have this much, but we don't know how much you have out there that we don't know about yet.' The bank people were real nice. That was an awakening, because this was the money she always, to the penny, had and now she can't keep up with the difference between a thousand dollars!"[23]

Fred reluctantly acknowledged that the confusing behavior of Mary—the smart, vibrant woman he had loved for half a century—scared him to consider what might follow. As I listened to his story, it reinforced an industry professional's[24] comment on caregivers' gradual recognition of their loved ones' prediagnosis symptoms.

"They notice that something's not right," she said, "a lot of times they can't put their finger on things." She noted family members notice their loved one:

- Can't remember
- Gets confused when driving
- Takes longer to respond when speaking

"So the forgetfulness…the something just isn't right, difficulty focusing and concentrating, are all things that they've mentioned."[25]

Beyond Fred and Mary's story, the other study volunteers would help me explore how caregiver gender or family relationship differences to the cognitively impaired family member might impact denial or awareness of prediagnosis issues.

* * *

George had passed away only three weeks prior to our meeting. Janice insisted that she'd be okay and thanked me when I told her she could ask to pause, reschedule, or simply decide to stop our interview if it became too upsetting. Because Janice was already attending a caregiver support group, she did not want the additional bereavement and counseling contacts I made available to each study participant.[26] George was nearly a decade older than Janice, who left her career to spend the last seven years to take care of him.

Janice said she had worked very hard and raised her children as a single mother, proud but without many luxuries. Her subsequent advancement into an executive position allowed her to cross paths with George, a successful business owner—and she was enjoying the attention, travel, and more financially secure lifestyle she had with him. "I learned to know him a long time before he invited me out. I loved the humor. I've always loved humor. By myself I'm not funny. I can't tell a joke, but I love humor and just the fact that we all had so much fun and that, and he finally asked me out about four months after that. But I knew him by then and I said, 'Yes.' On our second date he asked me to marry him, although I didn't know he was asking me to marry him. He said, 'I noticed you wear no rings.' I said, 'No.' Well, back then friendship rings were popular. He said, 'If I score you a ring, would you wear it?' I said, 'Yes.' I had no idea I was saying 'Yes' to marriage…we didn't get married for another year and by that time, I knew I wanted to be with him forever."[27]

However, Janice admitted it wasn't all laughter living with George, saying his self-confidence often served his business interests better than his family's. She thought his children probably believed they were always their father's second priority— first after his company and then later his second wife. So she didn't want to blame them for not trying to help when he was ill.

Janice paused briefly after sharing that the children had not been involved. I sensed she would speak more about that later but asked her to focus upon what initial signs there may have been to indicate that her husband was on a path to dementia. Janice said when she first saw minor changes in George's behaviors, she was more puzzled than worried. "My husband has always been very smart…just call out, 'How do you spell?' And he would just spell it…and it was always perfect. We had a great, big, thick dictionary—never pulled it out. Same way as far as history or knowledge: 'Well what river is that?' And he'd go, 'The Rhine River, the Amazon River,' always correct, so we never double-checked him. He was always correct. And… one day…I said, 'Oh, how do you spell?' And he said, 'I don't know.' I kid you not, I lifted my head and looked at him and said, 'You don't know?' And he said, 'No, I don't know.' And he acted like it didn't bother him a bit."[28]

Even as others mentioned him being different, she continued to believe he was responsible for whatever odd behavior he demonstrated. "I noticed that he would really repeat himself and my friend noticed it too. 'God, he's really repeating himself a lot.' I thought, 'Well, maybe it was the alcohol that night.' It wasn't. It was like he kept doing this."[29]

George's occasionally gruff personality also kept Janice from recognizing the early signs of his illness, because she thought he was just "acting like a jerk!"[30] As it got worse, it increased her anger more than her health concern. "The sequence was he started to behave oddly, in ways that were—like I said—arrogant, selfish, uncaring, extremely inconsiderate. It got to the point where I felt he was going to just grow to be an old, ugly, mean man—and I wasn't going to take it!"[31] Janice paused again, this time reaching for one of the tissues she had eyed upon sitting down. I told her to take as long as she needed and could see that part of her grief was in not forgiving herself for having judged him so harshly before his diagnosis.

Unbeknown to Janice, George had already begun losing his cognitive abilities. Although it had been frustrating to her, everything seemed in character—so she and others didn't recognize that he was covering.[32] In hindsight, Janice said, "I don't think he had any idea that he was covering up. He just would try to find ways to get things done because he could no longer do them. That didn't seem unusual to him. I remember one time he brought home a contract… and he asked me to read it for him. I had just gotten home from work also. I had a pretty big job myself. I said, 'You've got to be kidding. I'm not going to do that for you.' He didn't think anything of it. He just couldn't read it anymore."[33]

Janice paused for an extended moment, dropping her eyes to table while wringing her hands. "It's so gradual. It's so very gradual, but you don't really know that there's a memory problem. It starts out…Things that are out of character but, at first, I attributed it to being bored…and then something else would happen. I'd say, 'That's strange.' It was gradual."[34]

While Janice had been irritated by those strange occurrences, she said George's friends were perplexed. "He loved his golf. He just became, as I say, very confrontational at first. I mean, he'd accuse people of doing different things. 'Would you mind picking up my ball? I'm not going to play this hole.' He hit a bad shot or something, he didn't qualify it. The fellow would pick it up, and then he'd accuse him of doing something that he had no right to do. Of course, the short-term memory had gone. He didn't remember at that point that he had told this gentleman to pick up his golf ball. This is why it became confrontational."[35]

Janice finally realized that even if she didn't know what was wrong with George—things were not right. For her, that conclusion arose from her husband's peculiar cooking assistance. "I came home from work, and he had placed steaks in our hot tub to thaw them out! And I go out on the deck and…I said, 'George, what are you doing?'… He said, 'I'm thawing out the steaks.' Oh my gosh…So they're just floating in the hot tub! That's when I took him to a doctor."[36]

* * *

Alice pulled her gaze from the glass door to look directly at me. In a composed, but intense tone, she said she had not truly spoken to anyone about her own experience while taking care of her mother— not family, friends, coworkers, or even doctors. While self-educating herself on Alzheimer's, Alice visited a few dementia blogs and chat rooms, but had not become part of any caregiver support groups in her area. I felt it appropriate to remind her that all study participants' identities would be masked,[37] so she should feel free to share openly— as the university's Institutional Review Board protocol assured she and the others would have complete anonymity.[38] Alice's posture softened as she sat back into her chair without breaking eye contact. She told me when she read the caregiver research study's flyer[39]—she saw it as an opportunity for her story to possibly help others who might someday have a loved one diagnosed with Alzheimer's or other cognitive impairment themselves. I nodded encouragingly, and she began to reflect upon her five years as a caregiver for her mother, Audrey, and the years leading up to her assuming that role.

Her first thought was on how far off the family's perspective had been originally. "When we look back at it now, we understand that she was having symptoms years before we realized that's what they were…she wasn't paying her bills on time and things of that nature. We came to see that she had probably had it for several years prior."[40]

"Mom was the strongest figure in our life. She was the rock of the family, never let anybody down, and here she was. First, we thought she was messing with us because she would be a little bit of a jokester sometimes. We thought she was kind of messing with us."[41]

"Forgetting that she had plans to come to dinner with us— or always calling it 'the restaurant on the highway' versus 'Cracker Barrel'… I always thought Mom was just, 'Oh, she's being cute,' but it's probably she forgot the name of the restaurant… We went there once a week, but she couldn't remember what it was."[42]

Alice seemed disappointed that she hadn't deduced her mother's cognitive decline, especially given that her mother had been a caregiver to her father only a few years earlier. "It was easier to accept my father's dementia because my whole life he was sick… It was very hard accepting it, (for) my mother, because she was always the strong one, took care of my father, she always worked…she was always the matriarch and the strong one. I think I was trying to ignore it more with my mother."[43]

"She was always kind of absent-minded and she would lose her car keys…we just laughed, that was part of her charm… For the longest time I kept just saying, 'Oh yeah, that's my mother.'…I feel bad now…I think part of it was the thought that I didn't want to deal with, I tried to avoid it, and I, probably looking back, wish I had maybe looked into it with her sooner."[44]

"Friends were starting to call me and say, 'Things aren't quite right.' Call my mom up, and she's like, 'Oh yeah, I'm gardening today.' And, you know, say, 'Is Mom out gardening?' 'No, she's not gardening. She's not doing that.' And the neighbors…would say, 'We're worried about her.'"[45]

"In hindsight, the things like the…calls from her bill collectors and saying she wasn't paying her bills but she had plenty of money in the bank and she just was not paying them. Personal hygiene kind of took a back seat for her. Definitely cleanliness of the house."[46]

One of the household items Alice thought should have given them more concern about Audrey was an odd Thanksgiving incident. "Mother was living in her home and she called me and asked me if I had come down and put a pie in her spare refrigerator… (later) she showed me the pie that she had just made that day, and the pie that she found in her refrigerator…I know that both of them were made in her pie pans and that she had made both of them… I thought, 'That's a little unusual that she would bake a pie and then forget the next day that she had baked the pie, and bake another pie' but…we weren't looking for anything at that time."[47]

At another holiday gathering, Alice's brother and sister-in-law from out of state took Alice, her husband, their children, and Audrey to a "nice restaurant." While sitting there, she said Audrey looked at her own son, turned to Alice, and asked, "Who is that with Bill (Alice's husband)?" "I said, 'That's Mark, my brother, your son. He came into town and he is having lunch with us.' Mother looked at me and said, 'Yes, that's who I thought it was.' I knew that she had no idea…at that moment. Later that day she was fine."[48]

Whatever hopes Alice had been holding onto that her mother was merely experiencing some senior moments[49] and could continue to live on her own were finally dashed when "two men came to the front door offering to sweep up the leaves in the front yard…but they charged my mother over *a thousand dollars* for it, and she wrote the check and paid them…It was really clear that it was more than just forgetfulness or being too tired to maybe remember something, but there was something very wrong happening."[50]

The study's industry professionals' comments on caregiver gender matched the research literature that women are far more likely to assume the role within families than men.[51] To explore what factors might influence that decision, I asked Alice why she was the sibling who assumed the role of caregiver for their mother. "We actually moved down here a couple years prior to her diagnosis because when you would talk to her on the phone, she would seem so out of it, and when we got down here, we found out her original physician was just doping her up to…I mean like, six hydrocodone's a day. She was just doped up. So, the first thing we did when we moved here was take her away from that physician. Her new physician stripped all her medicines down and restarted and she got a lot better. So, we thought that's what we were looking at, was her growing old but healthier because we had gotten the medicines right."[52]

While she seemed comfortable with the decision they had made to relocate closer to her mother—in her continued response, gender appeared to be outweighed by adaptability. "We chose to move down because of all of my siblings, we were the most movable. With jobs that kind of necessitate that they stay there…So, of all…family members, we were the most relocatable… So we talked and we said we would move down here and make sure that Mom was doing okay. But like I said, we thought we were in for, 'she was on the wrong medicines,'…turned out to be totally different than that."[53] Beyond employment, other family circumstances solidified Alice's decision to look after their mother. "My sister was…going through a divorce. We didn't need to inflict this upon her children. It was easier for me to take the burden than to ask my sister."[54]

Alice seemed to hang on her last thought for a long moment before speaking again. She leaned in and seemed compelled to tell me, "I took care of Mother for probably five years before she died. Well I loved her, and—God just put me there to put her in my care."[55] "It was Alzheimer's…I was her primary caregiver…She chose to live in an ALF, an Assisted Living Facility.[56] In the beginning, that ALF was more of just an apartment that had services down on the first floor for her."[57]

Alice said she finally learned the basis for her mother's problems while on vacation when a neighbor called saying, "'You need to come home. Your mother doesn't know who she is or where she is!' We had her in the hospital for four days…She came home with us and then had another bad episode and they hospitalized her to—they actually Baker Acted her—she was claiming to the doctor that we were going to send her to the circus!"[58] Alice explained that an emergency room physician had overreacted to Audrey's touching his hand to "try to get eye-to-eye contact—he considered that assault and with the confusion and the assault they sent her to the behavioral sciences building there…for three days."[59]

Alice's face showed her frustration at the first doctor's reaction, but appreciation for another's—when she said, "The doctor that diagnosed her was the psychiatrist in the facility. He's like, 'She's not crazy, this woman has Alzheimer's.'"[60]

* * *

Yvonne's references to her mother, uncle, and sister seemed a bit muted, but her smile reappeared whenever she mentioned her grandparents. She spoke candidly about why she assumed the care-giver role instead of her grandparents' own children or in-laws. She said that her own mother was not well and that her uncle and his wife "were too involved with their careers, and I put mine aside.… You know, she reached out to me. How can I tell my grandmother, 'No'? She just kept on reaching out to me and wanting me to do for her, and I did. I just stepped in and took over, because I knew she needed help. I'm not going to turn my back on her."[61]

As her grandmother's health was failing, she agreed to become her grandfather's caregiver with no idea of the task that awaited her. "My grandmother had renal kidney failure. They were married for, like, 60 years. My grandfather and I were both caring for her with hospice, and she had mentioned things to me, 'Oh, he's getting really forgetful. I'm worried about Richard.' His name was Richard. 'I'm worried about him.'"[62]

"I didn't know anything about Alzheimer's. I didn't know any-thing about elder care. I was 25 years old. I would listen to her, and we'd kind of joke about how he'd come in the room and ask her if she wanted a cup of tea, and then leave the room and forget that he had asked her if she wanted a cup of tea, and she…never got her cup of tea."[63]

"I found myself as the granddaughter-daughter that was left there with my grandparents. There wasn't anybody else available to take on that responsibility…They raised both me and my sister. My sister lives in New York… I kind of felt like my grandparents had taken responsibility for us as grandchildren, that now it was kind of my turn to take responsibility to care for them."[64]

"As I was caring for her and we ended up having hospice in the home, me and my grandfather were both caring for her during her last weeks of life. She passed away together with us. So I still had an apartment, I was living on my own, working full time, but I had taken off time just to be with my grandmother as she was passing, and things like that. Then, she had said to me, 'I want you to watch out for him. He needs to go to the doctor and get this checked out,' and things like that. It was kind of like her last words to me, to really care about that. I told her, 'Yeah, I'll make sure he's all right.'"[65]

"I had a different relationship than most anybody else in my family did because of that dynamic of me growing up with him, so I was a little more protective…My sister doesn't have very much tolerance, so I would not have seen that as being a viable option and nobody else was around."[66]

Yvonne soon understood her grandmother's concern for Richard's memory. "He got lost driving. That was the first indicator."[67] Her smile reappeared when she said, "He used to take the dishes…out of the dishwasher and put them in the refrigerator. Then when someone said something to him, he would say, 'Oh, we need cold plates for salad.'"[68] She thought his living alone and grieving over his wife's passing was having an effect on him.

Someone opened and quickly closed the library conference room door, briefly disrupting our interview, but Yvonne was quickly re-engaged in her grandfather's story. I stayed in my researcher's observational mode and found myself intrigued by her sense of family responsibility. As she continued to talk about her grandfather's grieving, I learned that the strong, calming presence Yvonne offered before me had been forged by life challenges greater than her smile would suggest.

"He wasn't eating. He was losing his appetite. He would be confused about what day it was, and as time went on, I think…early on, it was hard for me to understand. There's a lot of things probably a year or so after my grandma died that were like…he would say, 'Where's my wife? Where did Gladys go?' That was a repetitive thing…She passed away in March, seven months later is when my mother died. My mother had come out to see her mom before she passed, and she was there the day before she died. She left to go back to Arizona, and then seven months later, my mother died."[69] Yvonne's face grew pale, then she said that her mother had been killed by a drunk driver, without elaborating—opting instead to return to speaking about her grandfather.

"One day, we were riding down the road…He looks off to the right and he says, 'That hospital over there, don't you ever take me there!' Well, this was the building that was the old Jefferson Memorial Hospital that had not been a hospital in probably 20 years…I actually worked in that building…My uncle worked out of that building, and he's referring to it as a hospital? I just busted out crying. I'm like, 'My gosh, he's been to the building when Uncle Joe and I both worked there. He knows'—'What is he thinking,' you know? I never, ever said, 'Well, Grandpa, you know that's not…' I never, ever, ever argued with him or debated with him, and thank God, I didn't. So, I just started crying, my grandfather—I just had tears running down my face, and he asked me what's wrong. I said, 'I'm okay. I'm okay, it's okay.' I said to myself, 'I've got to do something, I've got to do something.'"[70]

"It was horrific. Yeah, it was a terrible time. I was still working during that time period. I was working, so my grandfather was… alone. That was six months after my grandma died. Shortly after that, he had confusion about what happened to his daughter, Elizabeth, which to me was good, because he didn't remember that his daughter was killed. That's when it started becoming clear to me, 'This is a little bit more than grief and confusion.'"[71]

The Search for Answers

Fred said that Mary understood he was growing worried by her memory lapses, so she agreed to his accompanying her at her next doctor's appointment. "I was thinking something physical, so we went to the doctor's and had all the scans and the exams and basically was told she didn't have anything physically that was causing the problem. So, then we did a lot of testing through psychologist, and I don't remember all the specialties but, a lot of testing."

"At that time they said, basically she, like many people, have a memory issue, and they gave me a lot of things that we could do to help her with these memory issues. And so, it took a couple of more years before we really just determined, hey, this falls into the dementia program."[72]

Despite the exercise and nutrition recommendations, Mary's problems persisted—as did Fred's concern for her and his frustration with her doctors. "I knew there's a problem. 'What's wrong with her?' I would tell them about things she did, (things) she'd put up that we couldn't find or things that were lost. They all seemed to just take this as, 'Well she can pass the test.' 'I know, she's very bright. I kinda check her with things myself and she passes those tests, but she's not right! She's doing this, she's doing that. She forgets too much!'"[73]

He pulled his hands back to the kitchen table, when he realized they were excitedly flailing about as he spoke of his surprise that Mary's physicians had not given him the answers he was seeking. "Doctors are afraid that they're going to offend the loved one that brought them in there that said there's something wrong with them to start with, or offend the person who looks very much like you and I, while we're sitting here, at that early stage…'If I tell you that you've got dementia and that's gonna be a horrible disease, will you come back and see me next month?'"[74]

Fred's frustration fueled his drive for self-education, which led him to attend a local Alzheimer's caregiver support group with the hopes of learning what else he could do for Mary. Just as this study's industry professionals asserted, Fred found other dementia caregiver group members to be a vital repose of folks with similar experiences who listened intently to him and shared information on the resources and doctors they had been disappointed by or very pleased to find.

Eventually, Fred was successful in having Mary referred to one of the specialists mentioned at the Alzheimer's group. "When we saw him, he went through all the lab business and so on and so forth.

Then he said, 'How's everything else going?' to my wife. She said, 'Fine.' I said, 'It's not fine.' I think he suspected something right from the bat too. He performed the MMSE.[75] He didn't tell me the results, but I was there while she did it and I knew that she wasn't scoring very well on it. He immediately referred us to a geriatric psychiatrist. He performed the MMSE as well and gave us the diagnosis of dementia Alzheimer's type. I think by that time it was probably beyond the beginning stages."[76]

"They took an MRI and said, 'Yeah, she's got dementia, and her brain is shrinking.' He said, 'She's got dementia and Alzheimer's, and her brain is shrinking'…It would have been nice if the doctor would have took me to the side and not been in front of my wife. I thought it was terrible for somebody to do that…I wasn't mad, I just didn't think that was a thing to do, but she forgot it the next day. That's the way things are."[77]

"Okay, so now we've got the diagnosis. 'Now we've got a diagnosis, doctor. What are you gonna do?' He says, 'You take it like this and do this.' …We went through all of the dementia medicines and they all made her really sick, and then found out that the medicines that we were being given…were not the minimum medication that you might normally start. It was simply something that he had in the office that was a sample."[78]

* * *

George had reluctantly given in to Janice's insistence that she set up an appointment for him to see his doctor for a checkup with her at his side. "It was a family physician. She walked out of the room and came back in. Said, 'That's a nice shirt you have on,' and he said, 'Thank you, my son gave it to me.' She leaves, comes back in, and says, 'That's really a pretty shirt.' And he said, 'Thank you, my son gave it to me.' So, she just diagnosed him like that—with that!"[79]

Although she had previously spoken to the nurse when setting the appointment, Janice seized upon the opportunity to tell George's doctor about his odd behaviors. "The doctor was concerned and George was mad at me. I could just see steam coming. He was furious…and I turned to him and I said, 'Well, George, you do understand I had told you I was going to talk to the doctor about this.'"[80]

"The doctor could see how he was reacting. He hadn't said much, but you could tell he was greatly upset. The doctor said, 'Well, George, we're going to do an easy test on you.' She said, 'What I'm going to do is, I'm going to write you a prescription…It's your choice whether you take it or not and it's a very low percentage….(if) you choose to take it, you will notice a difference within two weeks…it's as simple as that. It's your choice.'"[81]

"Anyway, all the way home, he didn't speak to me…I went to the drugstore and I had it filled for him and I set it on the dresser. I said, 'It's like Dr. Hance said, it's your choice to try this and when you decide to, let me know and we'll see if it makes a difference.' It was probably a good week before he decided he would try it. I kid you not, within a week and a half he was back to his old self and it was a very dramatic difference for him. So two weeks later he came to me and he said, 'I apologize. I notice the difference in myself already.' I said, 'Well, I didn't want to say anything, but I noticed in a week and a half that you were back to your old self.'"[82]

Janice sounded very sincere and appreciative for Dr. Hance's manner of letting George become a part of the decision process. She spoke further about the doctor's insight and the medication regimen that followed. "She didn't really think that it was anything but dementia or memory problem. I call them the same because I don't really know that there is much of a difference. After they established that there wasn't a tumor or anything like that, that he was physically healthy, we did that and then I got him on his Social Security disability."[83]

"I had George on Namenda and Aricept, and I would say…I think these medicines, to a degree, hold them at a plateau, but the way I understand the medicine is, if you're at 100-point, and then 0-point is when you pass (away)—if you're not on medicine—you kind of go from 100 down to 0 at almost a straight line. If you're on the medicine, you stay at 100, 80, 70, and then when you drop, you're still back here. So, it might hold the cognitive ability a little bit longer but, ultimately, it doesn't do any good—but I'm glad I had him on it…If you can keep them at the 80, 70, 60—so you could still go out to dinner. He could not read a menu, but I'd say, 'Oh, over here…you like this dinner…you know you really like this,' and he would eat, and he would enjoy his meal. If he had not been on medicine, and if it truly dropped faster in the same amount of time, being alive, I might not have been able to do things with him. We'd go to the beach and look at the sunset. So, I think the medicine is worth it for a period of time. Then it comes to a point where it's not really doing any good, but I think, in the beginning, it helps. I think it helps."[84]

* * *

I could not discern whether Alice was more disappointed with herself or Audrey's doctors for not diagnosing her with a cognitive ailment prior to being Baker Acted. She assured me the family had looked into her problems before that incident, but with her earlier improvement following a revamping of her medicine—their suspicions went unresolved.

"I went to the doctor with my sister and watched the doctor give her the dementia test, and she…passed it. It was like, 'We know you shouldn't be passing this,' and it was very frustrating. We get back, and then that's when I had the conversation with my sister. I said, 'Well, you know, my physician…is just saying she will eventually fail this'…She said, 'I can tell you from a physician's standpoint, when you know they've got it and you can't prove it, it is very frustrating.' So we just came to a conclusion—it was frustrating…The frustration was in those months where you know something's wrong and you can't prove it. You know she has dementia, but they won't do anything about it because the doctors can't prove it. So you're in these months of total frustration. That's where the voices get raised, the things start happening that just…They're not normal."[85]

Alice recalled another item that may have signaled the end of her mother's independence. It occurred just before she received that disturbing call while on vacation. She said Audrey had been "taking the bus…for disabled seniors—they will come to your home, pick you up and take you to the doctor. They contacted me that she was no longer allowed to use it because they noticed when they dropped her off in front of the doctor's building, she didn't know what to do. They're not allowed to take you into the actual building. She was no longer allowed to use it."[86]

The diagnosis following the Baker Act incident, with the psychiatrist's exclamation that her mother was "not crazy," but instead had "Alzheimer's," answered many questions about Audrey—and spawned even more. "I was definitely prepared for the diagnosis. We thought she had it before we could get it proven. I don't know that there were surprises. There were—I don't necessarily want to call it a disappointment, it's a sadness."[87] "You know what the diagnosis is, you can see all the tests associated with it, then you have the observations and they're all consistent with it. It's deterministic in terms of how this goes. There's no off ramp. It's just a matter of how do you manage the process? And so, that was kind of the challenge to it for me. The hardest thing around it is just that you haven't done it before."[88]

"We made sure she got to all of her doctors' appointments. Towards the end, after the diagnosis came in and the mental thing had really become a big problem, we mostly used the house physician of the ALF, who was there every week, and that worked out well."[89] "They'd put me on speaker phone, so I was in the appointments with her…I had at least a monthly meeting with the company that was running the assisted living place where I would call in and we would sit, we would talk about what was going on, how was Mom doing, what was the care doing."[90]

Alice would go on to speak of Audrey's ALF care, the absence of her siblings, and her own constant visits bringing food and her mounting guilt at not being able to do more. Tears formed in her eyes as she told me how she watched her mother fall prey to her disease. "She was sitting in the chair reading the paper, or I thought she was reading a paper, but at a closer look, I saw that the paper was upside down. I said, 'Mother, what are you doing?' And she says, 'Just reading the paper.' I said, 'Well, you're doing trick reading, because you've got it upside down!' And my mother started crying and she said, 'But, you're very smart. Could you teach me to read? I could read one time, but I can't read anymore.'"[91]

I slid the box of tissues across the small table, and it took Alice a moment to collect herself before she offered another reflection. "She had some understanding. She was aware enough to know that she wasn't following everything. So I would say, in those early years, she really suffered greatly because she knew she wasn't totally right."[92] "She didn't know the diagnosis was Alzheimer's. She knew she had something seriously wrong and she knew she was losing her memory. We never told her and she never asked the diagnosis. If she ever heard it, she never remembered. She just knew she was losing her mind and losing her memory."[93]

* * *

Trying to keep up at work and look in on her grandfather in the months following her grandmother's passing, then her own mother's death—Yvonne found herself teetering between her own physical and emotional limits. "We brought in a caregiver to come in during the day, because I knew that he wasn't eating like he should, and he had lost weight. I knew all this—so this lady happened to have been a retired LPN.[94] She looked at me and she says, 'I'm going to tell you what's wrong with your grandfather, and you know you need to get him to a doctor. There could be something they could do to slow the process—I don't know.' She said, 'But, your grandfather, he has what they call either Alzheimer's or dementia.' I was like, 'Oh, my, gosh!'"[95]

Still challenged by her own grieving, Yvonne's heart was strained further whenever she returned from work and checked her home's answering machine. She said it, "Got to the point to where my grandfather literally was calling my house repeatedly, repeatedly. I kid you not, he would call my house probably 30, 40 times a day. Literally, one time I actually counted how many missed calls there was from him and it was 80! 'Yvonne, please call me. Yvonne, please call me. Yvonne, call me. Yvonne, call me. Yvonne, call me.' It was about the same thing, over and over...and whenever I would talk to him, it was pretty much, 'Somebody stole my coffee. I can't find this,' or 'This is stolen—my paper plates.' 'Grandpa, nobody's going to steal your paper plates.'"[96]

The work, the calls, the grief took their toll on Yvonne. "I, for the first time in my life, had anxiety.[97] I did not know what anxiety was. I knew something was wrong—I didn't know what it was. I literally called the doctor and …they prescribed something … After a while it did not work, then later I obtained a new PCP (primary care physician)."[98]

Yvonne said no one else in the family seemed concerned by Richard's growing confusion. However, things changed when her uncle asked her to suddenly leave work one morning to join him at her grandfather's house. "The day that he lost his telephone and he called my uncle, that's the day that my uncle realized, 'Okay, it's not him.' Up until that point, he just kind of kept his distance with everything. I think he honestly couldn't handle it because of having health conditions himself, but that particular day, though, he calls me. The police department was there, because he called and told them someone stole his phone. Back then, the police didn't even do anything about Alzheimer's dementia patients, I guess. So, anyways, I showed up there and I just put my mind together—thinking what he would do. I went, thinking of his little routines and stuff, and I go in the living room, then I go in the kitchen, and I go in his bedroom, look at the bedside, and then I go in the bathroom and look at the back of the toilet—there's the phone. Police department…couldn't find the phone. Uncle Joe couldn't find the phone. They'd already been there and searched the whole house. Nobody could find the phone. The battery was dead—couldn't ring it. I was like, 'Oh, here it is.' They were like, 'How'd you do that?'"[99]

Although her uncle did not offer further involvement, Yvonne realized she needed to push beyond her grandfather's resistance and finally get his doctor's professional opinion. "He had a wonderful primary care physician who is actually my physician now…They had already been going to him for years, so I think my grandmother, before I was part of the picture caregiving, my grandmother had talked with the doctor about her concerns about her husband. It wasn't an unfamiliar thing for that."[100] "It was hard to get him to go to the doctor. We go to the PCP and I tell him, I said, 'We have a caregiver and she's mentioned Alzheimer's dementia,' and I said, 'I really think there's something with that.'…and my grandfather goes, 'How dare you accuse me of losing my mind!'"[101]

Yvonne's lip quivered, as she seemed to relive her grandfather's unexpected scolding when she detailed their ride home. "This big ordeal in the doctor's office—I was bawling. Well, we get in the car. I'm crying and crying and crying, and he's just running his mouth at me…As soon as we hit the road, out of the parking lot, 'Honey, why are you crying?' Oh, my God, I just cried even more. I couldn't help it, and he's like, 'Please tell Grandpa what's upset you. Please tell me.' He said, 'I don't ever want you to be sad. You know I will do anything for you.'"[102]

Fortunately, her grandfather did not repeat his outburst, quietly allowing Yvonne to follow the directions of Richard's primary care physician. "He had us make appointments with the neurologist. At first they started looking at neuropathy, because he had some problems in his gait, and they were thinking it was something to do with, I forget what that—*this* is called."[103] Yvonne looked toward me and lifted her hand to her neck, briefly tapping her carotid artery. "Then they went through a whole bunch of questions. They had a whole thing that he was supposed to remember things. They asked him a bunch of questions with these picture cards and things like that, and then the neurologist did the brain scan."[104]

Yvonne moved her hand across the table to gently touch her grandfather's portrait. "He probably knew before the diagnosis came in, because…It was really sad. I can remember him sitting—he had a big easy chair, and he had a phone book. That was back when people had phone books—so he had a phone book in there, and there was all his friends from Pennsylvania, that's where they raised me—so we grew up there and a lot of their connections were still in Pennsylvania and friends that he had and things like that. He would look through the phone book, and he would sit there for hours with the phone book, and he'd say to me, 'I can't remember who this is.' I knew he knew he was losing his memory. He was at a point in the beginning where, as a man, he was aware that he was losing his ability to remember. That was probably the saddest part, to see him know what was going on. I think as the progression went on, it was good that he didn't have that struggle anymore. He just settled into life with Alzheimer's without knowing that he had it."[105]

The diagnosis clarified things for Yvonne, giving her some idea of what needed to be done next. She said, "They had started him on some medicine that was supposed to help slow down the progression. He had the type of dementia as well where there are many strokes throughout your life, and they show up like little dots on the scan. Eventually, it became obvious he couldn't be left alone after a couple of years, so I had to stop working or cut my hours back. I went through every stage with him, from being confused about the remote control and trying to make phone calls. At the end, I had a bed alarm on his bed, so (if) he got up in the middle of the night to wander—I'd hear the alarm go off. Basically stopped working and was 24/7 days a week for two years, full-time heavy duty caregiving, for the last couple of years."[106]

Who's with Me?

Fred retired from the business world long before Mary's challenges began, but his thought to assemble a reliable support network to help handle her illness echoed a project manager's team concept. "When she started to get much more symptomatic, I let my neighborhood folks know what was going on. A couple of them responded by saying, 'We thought there might be something like that.' They came out of the woodwork. 'My uncle had Alzheimer's' and 'My mother had Alzheimer's.' A lot of people were aware of what the situation was. The same thing was true with family and friends. Some of our dearest, oldest friends are still our dearest, oldest friends."[107]

His smile continued when he spoke of his family's involvement. "My daughter's a nurse...she's pretty knowledgeable about stuff... They live several hundred miles away—so it has to be something that happens in a phone call...Now my daughter's really involved in helping me with paperwork and so forth."[108] "She's real handy. She's been a big help to me...just backing me up. I would say, 'What do you think about this or doing this?' 'You know, that sounds good.'"[109] "My brother and his wife have been remarkable. They've been down to visit two or three times in the last couple of years. I brought them to the support group[110] meeting once or twice too."[111] "And another thing that really pleases me—Mary has one brother and two sisters, and they come every year without their spouses and spend three days with her."[112]

Fred started to speak about the grandchildren, then paused for a moment to choose his words carefully. His shoulders shrugged a bit as he said, "There's a period of time when you don't need Grandma. You liked them when you were little kids. We're kind of in that, 'We don't need Grandma and Grandpa' stage with them…I'm working on trying to get them down here next week for a visit, but it's tough. The two youngest ones are in Virginia. The older boys, I think they look of it as an obligation to be with her and say hello, but they don't want to get deeply involved. The younger ones, it's been, 'Well, why is it happening?' and 'What does it cause her to do?' and 'Does she know if I tell her this?' A lot of questions of what to do. I think it depends on the age, what they do."[113]

Despite his love of family, Fred explained why he never considered moving back—even though his daughter welcomed him to do so. "She's very well aware of what's going on. And I told her, when my parents got to the point where they couldn't care for themselves, I told them I wasn't going to bring them into my home based on what I saw it did to friends when they brought their parents in—it cost them their marriage! I said, 'I'm not going to put that burden on our daughter. We will figure out a way of caring for ourselves. You can come and visit anytime.'"[114]

Fred believed the most important member of his team was actually Mary. Anything he or the others might do would be directed by her abilities or changing needs. He wanted to speak to her as his wife—not a patient, for as long as was possible. Fred said he told Mary how he felt once they finally had a diagnosis from the doctors. "So I go home. I say, 'Well Hon. We got some bad news. Maybe bad news, maybe not so bad news. But it's not good news. You have been diagnosed with what probably is an Alzheimer dementia. But…we know a lot about this disease. It could've been you have been diagnosed with a very aggressive cancer—you're gonna die in six months…you could've had a stroke and been in a wheelchair. But you're diagnosed with a disease that's going to be not good—if you live long enough. But here we are 75 years old—who knows how long we're gonna live? So I choose, and I hope you will choose, that we will live this disease as if it's not a disease to be ashamed of. We'll tell your friends. We'll tell the children. We will tell the world. We'll tell anybody… "Oh, I have dementia. If you see me do something wrong, I have dementia."' I said, 'And I think, we will just maybe, because you're in good health, we might just outlive this disease before it gets you and takes over you. One of these other bad things might happen. But between now and then, we're gonna be the happiest couple that anybody knows.'"[115]

The non-family portion of Fred's team included an actual support group for caregivers dealing with Alzheimer's- and dementia-afflicted loved ones. "A friend of mine…says, 'You need to get to a support group.' There were days I'd say, 'This is really tough dealing with a mental illness.' I wouldn't get much sleep. Anyhow, so I took (the) advice…and it was wonderful. I could not say enough."[116] Fred then followed his support group's advice in seeking respite[117] to stave off becoming too worn out by his caregiving duties while Mary was still at home. "The church has a program called 'Higher Helpers.' I used that two days a week. Hospice[118] has a program with a volunteer. I used that one day a week. Then I used the neighbors for shorter periods…to run and get something real quick in the daytime. I have four, five neighbors that would come over and stay with her briefly. I didn't feel like I could burden them very long so I used that."[119] "The big thing for me was not to mess up the head with trying to do everything, but to get away. Again, I learned that by going to meetings and reading. They call it, you need 'your quiet time,' or 'your away time.' Now, when I first started that two to three hours was, 'Okay, I'll go get all these things done.'"[120] Fred said eventually he used respite to just "go out and have a cup of coffee with a friend and talk for a while, or go to the library or go sit at the pool and just relax and let your mind clear…There's a tremendous difference in what goes in your head when you know you're responsible for the person and when you know there's someone else that is filling in that responsibility for a short period of time, and that makes a big difference I've found."[121]

Because Fred had learned of this research study from a caregiver support group facilitator, I asked him to elaborate more on why he and the others attended group meetings. "Many of the people that come here, their spouse is in the early stages, and the first week we go through a list of documents—'Do you have these? If not, get them.' 'Who's going to make decisions for you, the caregiver, if you go to the hospital?' Most married couples have their spouse doing it. Your spouse can't do it, maybe she can do it today, or he can do it today, but in a year, they probably won't be able to do it. 'Who's going to be your health surrogate?'…'Have you talked to your kids, besides the legal documents?' 'Have you talked to the kids of what your wishes are compared to what they think you should do?' One of the stories you hear over and over, kids have one idea, parents have another idea, and they haven't talked about it. So when the crisis comes, they're in a clash of, 'What do we do with Mom?' or 'What do we do with Dad?' So, talk about those things…'What is your problem that you're dealing with right now?' Then they hear suggestions from others, or maybe, 'Go read this book' or that sort of thing to get an idea. That's kind of the natural thing that we do."[122] "One of the comments you hear at the support group meetings here is, 'After a while, there are no longer any surprises, there are only disappointments.' That's the absolute truth. They also say, 'Don't wait too long before you get help—professional help.' Of course, everybody does…I think a number of the folks that are involved in the group now are taking those steps much sooner than they otherwise might. Having in-home companions like housekeeping. Things like that."[123]

Fred would later detail the issues leading to his inability to continue caring for Mary at home, but her change of venue from home to facility appeared to also shift his ongoing participation role at the support group. "I think it's very helpful because I get some great feedback from them. I know that some of the information that I can provide is doing them some good. I know that the information that I received early on did me a great deal of good."[124] Encouraged by my attentive nodding, he continued, "I realize that no one can go through it alone. No one can go through it without having some advance information about the likely change. It doesn't always occur. Each patient is different, but I know how important that was for me. I think it's that important for the ones that are coming on, earlier on, in the journey. It makes me feel good. I get a great deal of satisfaction out of it. I see some of the folks here who have lost their loved ones over the last few years, who, after some hiatus you might say, came back and took training as facilitators and they're now running meetings and so on. I'm not quite ready for that yet."[125] I silently noted to myself that it would be interesting to learn if, after Mary's passing, Fred himself would become a caregiver group facilitator—and if he did so for bereavement or to add a special purpose for their Alzheimer's journey.

* * *

I first met Janice when I had been an invited guest to recruit study participants at the caregiver support group that she attended.[126] The group consisted of a dozen people bonding together to help each of them progress along similar caregiver paths—some with a loved one currently in the throes of a dementia, most with Alzheimer's, others now the survivor of one recently departed. Knowing this, I hoped I did not show my surprise as she recalled her first visit to a caregiver group—which she decided not to join shortly after George was diagnosed. "They were all white-headed little old people, little old gray people. We were still…(significantly)…younger than most of them."[127]

Next to make a disappointing first impression on Janice was an online caregiver group. "All types of caregivers would get on there— extremely good caregivers, extremely selfish people. I remember one young woman—she was just worried about her sex life. I mean, this blew my mind! That all she was worried about was him not being able to service her anymore is basically what it came down to! How do you—now, this is a conversation that's in view of *two thousand* people. There are people jumping on, 'Oh yeah, I know just what you mean.' I'm saying, 'Hey, wait a minute. We need to keep some sanity here or some perspective of, hey, let's not feel sorry for ourselves. This is the person who is dying, not you!'"[128]

Whether my poker face needed work, or Janice was simply embarrassed by her own words, she admitted her state of mind was not good when George was first diagnosed. "Just a total loss. Knowing I was gonna lose him…He took care of everything—finances, groceries. He was in control, and I liked it. I didn't want it…I'd done that. I'd been married before, raised two children, worked hard, and he took care of me."[129]

George's diagnosis also forced them to sell his business, amid a myriad of lifestyle changes for them both. "I knew that…He wanted his children, who are now adults with their own families, to come, on his terms, to Florida to take care of him. They weren't going to uproot themselves to come take care of a father who was, at best, disruptive in their lives. They were very young when he left, when she (George's first wife) kicked him out I should say."

Instead, Janice decided to prepare for the long haul on her own and take care of him at home. "I was young. I felt I could do it…I bought a house big enough with a pool, so I'd be happy knowing that I'd be stuck there for, in my mind, maybe 12 to 18 years. I bought a house that I knew I could be happy in with my surroundings."[130] "We had been married…So, in my mind, I had made a commitment, in sickness and in health…As hard as it was, and it was hard, it was very hard—I did move all the knives, all the scissors, I took the knobs off the stove—I made the house as safe as I possibly could."[131]

Janice found a home near George's sister—and she gratefully welcomed her to visit them every day. Janice's own children "told me to turn to them, call them and vent,"[132] but compared to his sister, the others were far less supportive. "My family was pissed at me because they didn't like this. They didn't like him…There was a lot of…My friends all said, 'Oh, you're doing it just for his money.' They didn't—I don't know. Nobody—Anyway, that's what I did."[133]

Things were even worse with his children. "They were brutal. They were just brutal."[134] I listened as she rationalized their behavior while constraining her disappointment they weren't there for George when he was helpless. Janice said she believed that from his children's perspective, George "'…had failed as a husband, failed as a father.' Yet, he provided for them, took care of them."[135]

She stared at the table and said what she believed had been the rest of the family's mind-set even after she left her job to care for George at home. "I think that when people measured it out, versus finances and living…I think that they would rather have seen him just go and not be alive."[136]

We shared an extended pause as she reached for another tissue. While Janice appeared to quietly reflect upon her last words, I noted how her somber tone and ugly characterization of their blended family's perspective fit with a comment from one of the study's industry professionals. "Unfortunately, stressful situations are times when old past hurts of previous divorces, and blended marriage, and relationships, and things like that kind of surface. They might have put them aside, but now they kind of come to light again, which impacts their ability to think clearly and stay focused on the needs of everybody involved."[137]

Janice tried to accept the caregiver role she took on as best she could, but admitted the strain and George's own frustrations directed her back toward an outside source of support. "Well, I hid something on him. He couldn't find his shoes, which I must have moved. I mean, it was just small things. Nothing drastic. It was just little, tiny things that didn't amount to a hill of beans as far as I was concerned. To him, it was a giant thing that had happened. He accused me of taking his keys. At that point, I would argue with him because I wasn't into the Alzheimer's."[138] "It made our personal relationship very difficult to the point of—I just couldn't accept it. I was putting my head in the sand, so I would get angry and think, 'I can't live with him anymore. He's angry about everything.' So I came to counseling here, and Christine said to me, 'Let's start from the beginning. How do you feel about your husband?' And I said, 'I love him dearly.' She said, 'That's where we'll start.'"[139] "I learned that I was not alone. That everybody else had similar problems, not always the same, but similar situations. That you just do not confront them. You either change the subject, or you agree with them and say, 'We'll take care of it.' Don't be confrontational at all—none of that which I was doing. We would get into heated arguments. Then, he'd come and apologize. Then I would apologize."[140]

Given her earlier decisions not to participate in a support group, it was interesting to hear what had changed her mind. "I knew that if I get frustrated, go for somebody. Go talk to somebody. So, I looked it up online. I saw there was an Alzheimer's Family Organization,[141] and they had support groups. So, I went to several because timing was always difficult. So, they have one at 6:00, they have one at 10 in the morning, different ones. So, I would try different ones, and so many of them, they only had one person, or just the leader, and it was fine. I mean, it served the purpose, but I stumbled upon the one that had more people, and I didn't want to just go in and complain about my situation. I wanted to be educated, and the one that I go to, she's very good about finding things, printing out—Letting us talk, yet giving us some direction…The first couple of meetings, it was scary…They tried not to overly scare you or give you too much at once, but to realize that this isn't going to go away. It's not going to get better. It's going to come in waves. Some will be a little bit better, and then a dip, and then a little bit better, and then a dip."[142]

"We used the analogy, 'It's like swiss cheese.' If you get a whole pack of sliced swiss cheese, there may not be any holes, but when you peel one away, there's some holes there. When you peel another one away, there's some holes, and so, one day things might seem okay, and another day…"[143] The group leader's teaching and the other caregivers' genuine understanding and concern for her situation helped Janice to cope better—even though it did nothing to halt the disease's progression.

She spoke candidly about her later enlightened perspective as a caregiver to a cognitively impaired family member. "If you don't look at the whole picture and think this is how I have to handle this—I can't change this, but I can change this…If you do that, then you can deal with it better. Like I know George is gonna have a bowel movement in his underpants and he's gonna pee all over his shorts every day because he tries to go to the bathroom—that's not gonna change. I'm not gonna get angry over it. That's what you have to learn. You can't get upset over the little things. You have to get upset over the big things."[144]

* * *

Alice said she did not want to be ignorant about her mother's illness, so she began to self-educate on Alzheimer's and dementia. "I just read anything I could—articles, books, read whatever I could get my hands on to learn about it, and then there is a new gentleman on *YouTube*…and he has a mom that has Alzheimer's and he does *YouTube* videos that I watched every week. It's nice to see other people kind of going through what you're going through because you know everyone talks about it, but it's not really out there, so you actually see. So it was very nice to watch him interact with his mom and stuff, so I watched his videos all the time as well."[145]

I noted that within Alice's caregiving experience, her self-reliance may have been a reoccurring factor in her actions, and possibly behind her not having opened up to others before our interview. After a quick glance through the glass office wall, she continued. "The people at my office who are closest to me knew that it was going on, were there for me if I wanted to share things, but were kind enough not to pry…There was a variety of different ways that they dealt with some of it…the 'Suck it up and get over it' type of thing…which, in some cases, was helpful and, in some cases, was not."[146] "The only thing I was aware was the hospice support—I mean, hospice support group. For me, I don't feel that talking really helps. I mean, talking is not going to help unless they are really willing to help. For me, it was more time."[147] "I did go to grief counseling at a hospice after she passed away. I had a friend and my cousin who knew what was going on, but they all agreed that I was doing too much and I always agreed that I wasn't doing enough. We never came to an agreement on what I should be doing."[148] "I was not even on the Facebook…I just didn't want to do anything. I hate when I have to tell people what I'm doing because I feel I am getting their sympathy or getting like, 'Oh, wow.' I hate when people say, 'Wow, you are doing this?' I don't like that because I'm not doing it to hear wows. I'm not doing it to get pity. I don't like talking to people. I just stopped socializing because I don't want to tell anybody what I'm doing."[149]

Her gaze dropped, as Alice listened to her own voice reflecting on herself, to herself—temporarily oblivious of my presence. "Over a five-year period, I was becoming less social. 'I don't want to go to any parties. I don't want to socialize anymore. I don't want to talk to people.' I just am like that now. I hesitate going to social gatherings. I don't like somebody coming to my house—family is fine. I'm not a social person anymore. I would not like to talk. Some people probably get support…if I had support, maybe I would've loved it, chatting on the phone…but that's what…changed my life."[150] She lifted her eyes slightly, offering a hint of why Alice may have agreed to become a part of the research study. "So my advice for anybody would be, 'Don't let it change your life. Find a way to continue.'"[151]

Once Alice's introspective moment had passed, her self-reliant tone reappeared. "I had the help of my minister and the very, very small church I belong to, so there was some support there…With the help of…people that I met down here—the church, the psychologist, the various professionals, my husband—I had the support that I needed."[152] "I didn't really burden my husband with it either. We didn't talk about it, like what was going on or how much was being spent for this or that or how much money was there, whatever. I was just, 'Really, don't worry about it…we're not going to be financially liable for it, so just don't worry about it.' We had small kids. We had our own things that he was very focused doing so it wasn't necessary for him to be engaged in it."[153]

From our interview alone, I could not deduce whether Alice's caregiver self-reliance affected, or was affected, by her description of the out-of-area siblings' involvement. "They would be very willing to help financially—emotionally they were not there."[154] "One sister called very frequently. My other sister and my brother called very infrequently and my conversations with them usually revolved around, 'Hey we're trying to call Mom. She's not answering.'"[155] "My brother's not an emotional person at all. Never thought to call my mother ever and just to say, 'Gee, Mom, how are you doing?' Never. Never."[156] Alice said her brother "knew what she's dealing with—very factual, very factual, never, never dealt with it at an emotional level at all. That was my job. One time my husband actually sent an e-mail, because my brother is not one to call or not one to talk between visits. Months would go by. He actually sent my brother an e-mail and he said, 'It would be nice if you called your sister. She's not dealing well.' He actually called and I was so surprised that he called out of the blue to see how I was doing, and then afterwards I said something, 'Did you put him up to this?' He admitted it. I mean, that was my brother. He's still that way."[157] With widening eyes, Alice recalled her most shocking sibling call. "My one sister called me up and said, 'I need my inheritance now!' I was like, 'What are you talking about? There is no inheritance! There's Mom's money and it's Mom's money until Mom passes away. I don't have a crystal ball—her mom lived to be 95 or something like that. I don't know what medical things are around the corner—I don't know how long this is going to take. There is no money until, you know, whenever.'"[158]

Still shaking her head at her sister's call, Alice said she was grateful that her parents had been somewhat prepared financially. "I was very, very fortunate in the fact that I faced absolutely no financial issues with this, because my father was a wizard, if you will, with finance. He had saved a tremendous amount of money and left it so that we could take care of Mother. It was no trouble whatsoever. We didn't have to worry about which ALF to pick. We could pick the most expensive one…When we chose the place, Mother was pleased with it. I just told the person, 'Look, what's the best setup you've got?' They said, 'We've got this thing on the top floor that's actually a two-bedroom, all sorts of setup.' I said, 'Sign her up,' so we did that. That was very fortunate. We were able to provide all of the things."[159]

Alice continued, "It was her money and that was very clear, I think. That was another thing that you've got to keep in your head, 'It's not your money, it's her money. You're just distributing it for a while' and so don't ever get this idea of, and I think it's possible, people might, 'I don't want to do this 'cause it's gonna cost this much money and they don't really need it,' or whatever. It was always anything that I could think of to do. Buy a new TV for Mom, a new couch, a chair or you know…whatever it could be. 'Yes, we're gonna do that.' 'Hair appointments every week,' right? 'To get her nails and her hair done,' right? To just look nice. Things like that. Yeah, do you have to do those things and, 'Does it cost money?' 'Yeah, but it's her money,' and I know that she would like that, 'So that's what we do.'"[160]

Once again, Alice credited her father's foresight in preparing for their illnesses. "He was very good at managing his funds and he knew how much it would cost. He said eventually this would happen…and this is where the money is."[161] "She did have a long-term care policy,[162] for a three-year long-term care policy. I told my brother and sisters we needed to do this…One said, 'Well, you know, what if she lives longer than three years?' I said, 'Well, if she lives longer than three years, we'll pay at the end of the three years,' but I said, 'We need to use that up.'"[163] "We agreed, 'Do whatever it is that's necessary to take care of Mom. If it means that we spend *every dime*'—that my mother had, my siblings were on board…if it meant we spent *every dime*, then that's what we needed to do. That didn't happen."[164] "The biggest thing here was that it was never a financial burden…because…there was enough there. You weren't sure, especially at the start, 'cause you start looking at, it's *ten grand* a month! You know, you start realizing, 'Holy crap, this is $300 a day!' And you start doing the math on that and start thinking about it and it's pretty scary but as her health started to decline, it became apparent that the money was going to outlast the life. Sadly, that actually takes stress off of the conversation."[165]

* * *

Yvonne's recalling the totality of the caregiver responsibilities she handled over 15 years ago brought an astonished look to her face. "I had to start taking over paying the bills and finance things. I had to start taking over all of his medicine, providing everything for the household that he needed, his care, dressing him, bathing, cooking, cleaning. It was just, one thing would be done and then another thing would come up. I've never been a mother, so I'm sure mothers go through the same thing in a different way, but for me, as the caregiver, it was a little overwhelming, for sure."[166] Astonishment gave way to perspective as she continued. "I think the vigilance that it requires to be a caregiver, like you're kind of always on duty, so I didn't really process a lot of the grief of the death of my grandmother and Mom, because I became a full-time caregiver very quickly. I think a lot of that came afterwards. It really hit me hard, but during that time, I don't think I could have done it without the support of my friends who were like family." Yvonne smiled brightly again. "They prayed with me and they listened to me and they offered suggestions and encouraged me to make sure I was taking breaks. That was new to me. I didn't understand that, but when I understood, 'Okay, yeah, I need to do these things so I'm a better caregiver.' Then it was like, 'Okay, I could give myself permission to go do something fun,' because the responsibility was so overwhelming."[167]

"I didn't understand introducing other people into caregiving, so that he could get used to them and not be confused. I learned that's better to do that really early on. I was a safety blanket to him. We had such a really tight relationship, because we cared for his wife, my grandma, while she was dying, together. That bond was there. His peacefulness was associated with my presence being around, like his sense of comfort and safety and all that kind of stuff…I had a beautiful church with some beautiful people there that volunteered to come over and give me a break…I would go to the park…I'd go grocery shopping, or I'd go take a nap somewhere…they were like family to me. Some older women would come and stay with him and give me a break. Another lady who's still my friend…she's a minister, and she would come, like when I went to go bury my mother in Arizona. He couldn't be left alone at that point, and she stayed there for a week with him. She kind of adopted him as her grandpa because she never really had a grandpa, so we became like a little family. We've bought each other Christmas presents and things like that. It was a really beautiful time."[168]

"I also went to a drunk-driving bereavement group seven months after my grandma died, when my mother died. They taught me a little bit more about self-care,[169] because a lot of what that focus was, was processing your grief and going through that. I was really thrown—my biological mother passed, and…my grandmother who raised me, who was my mother, had passed. Then I was caring for my grandfather who had Alzheimer's, so I was thrown into a kind of a whirlwind."

"I think the job that I had at that time…there was a beautiful lady named Jackie there and she says that, 'I signed you up for the drunk-driving bereavement group.' She knew my grandpa. I was still working, so he was at the beginning of, 'Oh, I don't know how to work the microwave,' and he'd call me at work and say, 'How do I work this?' Because I would prepare meals and he would stick them in there. I think she saw where I was at, and encouraged me and just basically told me, 'You're going to this support group when you're taking time off work.' I never ended up going back to work, but I went to that support group, and really found an outlet and encouragement to do self-care and make sure I could take care of myself to take care of my grandfather, sort of thing."[170]

Yvonne's peaceful demeanor, as she described a change in her life's priorities, seemed in great contrast to what she'd depicted shortly after her grandmother died. She nodded and said, "That transition was right when my mother died, so the lady that I worked with had said, 'I don't want you to worry about work right now. Go to the bereavement group, take care of your grandfather,' and I just never went back to work after that."[171] "I saw firsthand how those support groups change people's lives. Just having somebody to vent to just relieves some of the stress. Not all of it, but some of it. Knowing that you're not alone, that's priceless."[172] "I moved out of my apartment. I think I held onto it for a while, and then I let go of it, and I pretty much moved in with him full time within the first two years. I think it was pretty early."[173]

"Once he became my responsibility, I didn't realize that I would have that passion. It just all hit me one time. Like, 'Oh, my God. He took you in. Now you're—It's role reversal!' I just took it very seriously for him. I took everything…in his life extremely serious. …That surprised me, that I would be able to…I didn't realize that I would take it on like he was my child, like I had that mothering protection over him."[174] "It was the hardest thing I've ever done, the most challenging. I was tired all the time, especially near the last three or four years, because he would get restless at night and things like that. It was extremely difficult. I went through it earlier in life, because my grandparents raised me, so he was my father, but he was my grandfather."[175]

"I think I was really blessed. My grandfather had provided and saved for his later years. Otherwise, it would've been impossible for me to be a caregiver. He had a pension…He had a certain amount of his health care that was allotted towards home health aide and things like that. He never told me about it, so I had to find it. Wish I had found it earlier. I wish it was laid out a little bit clearer, like he had had things written down, because I could've utilized it earlier on, that resource, but I did and made the most of it in the last three years, I think. That was hard."[176] "Later we found out he would have benefited from VA benefits, because my grandfather served in World War II. Yeah, so we knew nothing about that, so he paid cash. It was paid for. He was blessed. He had finances for all that. So, no, none of that was never ever an issue. Thank God, because I realized… that is a huge issue and it affects a lot of families because of trying to find somewhere and getting help from the government, vice versa. I realized that."[177]

Yvonne had characterized her friends as family, but said her uncle and sister both had some unresolved issues with Richard. "He had a son that lived maybe ten minutes from him and had not been to see him, had not seen him in…years. He decided once I took over, he was just considered dead to him because he was not going to deal with the things."[178] With Yvonne's mother absent, then deceased and her uncle self-detached, her remaining family consisted of her out-of-state sister and a local nephew. "She didn't contribute to anything, but when he passed away, he wanted to leave everything to me. She still doesn't know this, but I told him, 'No. You have to split everything with her,' so he did do that." Yvonne leaned in to say, "He was actually very abusive growing up, so I don't fault my sister for not being there. I don't hold that against her. She was very supportive in the way that she knew how, and she did come out and see him before he died. That was good. He told her he was proud of her, and they sort of made amends… I had dealt with that previously to my grandmother dying…I had spent a lot of times in prayer about certain things of my life, and I worked through those issues…I understood she wasn't capable emotionally or mentally to step up to the plate, and she had unforgiveness issues towards him. That was all part of my understanding, but I do wish she would've been more involved, or at least checked in to see how things were going."[179]

"My other relative, who was alive and could've been available to help, my nephew, was stealing things. Then I had to deal with that. There was a time that was probably five years into taking care of him that somebody had called elder care services. He was in the hospital. The man came, and he's doing his job and he's interviewing my grandpa and he's checking me out and looking at the whole situation. At the end of the interview, he said to me, 'All I can say to you is—no good deed goes unpunished,' and he says, 'It's confidential. I can't tell you who called, but as an investigator, one thing that I do is ask myself, "Why is this person calling at this particular time?"' I don't know for sure, but I think it was my nephew that had done that. It was just something kind of ugly that a relative could have helped, and I was doing everything I knew how to do to provide and care for my grandfather and take on that role. That family would do that is actually still painful to think about. Yeah, so that's why my friends were more a true family than family. It was so hard. I wish that my nephew would have helped and not hurt the situation."[180]

Reality Altered

Sounding like he was speaking to a new member of his Alzheimer's support group, Fred tried valiantly to point toward a positive item along a bleak horizon. "If there's any good thing about this disease, at all, is it gives you time to work into it. It's not like a heart attack or stroke…This builds up slowly and you kind of go with it—and the support groups have been very helpful—and the main thing is, you go into their world, they're not going to go in your world."[181]

Fred was prefacing his comments on learning to adapt as Mary's reality was altered. "That's why I actually wanted to get a power of attorney signed and everything before she was actually diagnosed. I understand once they're diagnosed, they're not legally able to sign any legal documents…(the attorney) asked her some questions and she was still cognizant enough to answer." He said they were very fortunate she could still sign, "the durable power of attorney,[182] not just the power of attorney. Durable power of attorney."[183] "We had never discussed anything like this. Never… After she was diagnosed…I went back to Mr. Mueller. He re-did the stuff again, basically putting everything in a trust which we'd had anyhow…but with me as a sole trustee, our kids as the successor trustees…We applied for Medicaid[184] and that was awarded in March of 2015—I think it was. That made a hell of a difference."[185] "I don't have any IRA's or trust fund or anything like that, and we were able to get her on Medicaid on the first go around. It only took like three months and I've heard some horror stories that it sometimes takes a year or so. But what is great is it goes back to the time you apply—rather than when they approve it. So that's a great thing. So we were very fortunate in being able to get Medicaid. The drawback to that is, only a few facilities accept Medicaid patients anymore. 'Oh the *Garden View Residence*…that's a nice facility.' 'No, we don't take Medicaid, but we'll keep her here for $8,500 a month.' I said, 'Okay, when I hit the lottery I'll come back to see you.'…A good half of them that I called and checked with…what I thought the nicer places, more room and more things to do—and not that she can do anything now, but you know at the time. None of those would accept Medicaid, so it was very selective. Plus having a Medicaid facility that has a lock down.[186] So, we had to settle for one that…and I'm not criticizing them. They are doing a nice job, but they don't have quite as many amenities that some of the other places have, but she still gets decent food and decent care and she gets some physical therapy and some play time."[187]

Fred scanned my face, perhaps searching for a sign of judgment because he told me Mary was on Medicaid. My expression never altered, but I knew the subject can cause stress for those pursuing it or generate contentious conversations in both the public and professional arenas. I wondered what Fred would have thought of my own practitioner-scholar objective for sparking a broader discussion on the topic within the financial planning profession. I already knew that interest would once again have to wait, as my current research priority was this caregiver study book project. Only a few months earlier, I withdrew a working paper, *Medicaid Millionaires: The Ethics of Evasion*,[188] from an academic conference to prioritize two others, as all three had been independently accepted for poster presentations.[189] No judgment was made by me or sensed by Fred, and his next comment came slowly, heavy with a reluctant acceptance. "Even though my wife's in a facility, I can't do anything about that, but I know she's well taken care of. It's a relief to me to know that she is, and they do call if there's an incident or a problem or anything. As I say, I try to make sure they all know I'm there."[190]

I asked Fred how things began to change when he started to care for Mary at home. He said papers, keys, cooking utensils, and other things would just disappear. "You had to watch her all the time. She had a big thing in hiding stuff…She used to save money that way. She would hide stuff in a book or in a particular pocketbook or stuff like that. When she went into the facility…she'd been down there two weeks, and…my daughter is sitting in the kitchen chair and we have an extra pillow on all of the chairs, and the cat was in the chair and jumped off the chair, scooted the pillow. She raised the pillow and here's her baby picture under the seat. So I thought, I better check some of these other pillows. And most of the pillows are sewn in, but in the living room, there's a loveseat that doesn't have pillows. I picked up the loveseat and here's an envelope with about $15 worth of change in the envelope… And a couple of years ago, I was sorting through some of the books. She went to Weight Watchers for a while and the Weight Watcher menu box—I was going to get rid of that and my daughter said, 'Let me just see if there's any recipes in there that I would like.' So she was going through the box and found ten, $100 bills—*a thousand dollars* in the recipe box! So we went through everything then. All the old pocketbooks, clothes, anything we could think of where she could hide money. She was very good at hiding money."[191]

"I found some money, one time, under the mattress in the spare bedroom. My grandson said that he thought that some of his money was missing, and I just gave him the money back. I said, 'It might have been her, I don't know.' I don't know whether he might have spent it, but it doesn't make any difference. It was gone, and I don't want my grandson to have to pay for anything he doesn't have to. He understood."[192] Fred also said it wasn't until after he had already replaced his own "missing" driver's license that he found it, "tucked away in the bathroom."[193]

Yet a bigger challenge than her hiding things was his wanting to reason with her. "The weakness we have as caregivers, we are thinking of them as how they used to be, rather than where they are. So, when she wouldn't agree with me, my deal initially was to argue and convince her. She quit doing everything in the kitchen somewhere along the way. One day I made lunch. I said, 'Lunch is ready. Come in for lunch.' And she just sat there. So I said, 'It's going to get cold. You need to come in and eat now.' And she just sat there. And I said, 'I want you to come in the kitchen right now! We're gonna eat!' I could see she was starting to get upset. And that was a very trivial thing, but I let my emotion…and that was the early stages. I would let my emotion take over rather than just being calm, and then she would get emotional and be even more negative in what she was going to do."[194]

"I worked in supervisory and management positions all my life. I was used to giving commands to people, or direction, if you want to say it nicely, and I would expect them to do it. Doesn't work with an Alzheimer's or dementia person."[195] Fred said he learned it was his adjusting to Mary's momentary state of mind that affected whether or not he could communicate with her. "One day…she didn't want to put on a particular blouse that I had gotten out for her. I said, 'That goes with your pants.' And all the reasons why you should do it. And she just was fighting, 'No!' I felt myself getting mad so I went out of the room, and this is where I learned that—went out the room. Calmed down. Came back. When I came back in, I said,

'Let's talk about what just happened.' She said, 'What happened?' I said, 'You didn't want to put that blouse on.' 'No, I'll put it on.' That was the point where I realized that the logic that we used for years and discussing, resolving issues, didn't work. And so now, it's diversion and go back to it later on."[196] Fred added, "The other thing I've learned, they learn how to read emotion very quickly. So, you can say the right things but if your emotion doesn't tell them that, and if your facial expression doesn't say that, they know that's not what you're saying."[197]

Fred and Mary lived in an active retirement community that offered playing cards, golf, dances, music, and dinner outings. "In the several months after the diagnosis, maybe even a year or two, we still maintained a lot of the same contacts. It finally got to the point where she didn't want to go anymore. That was another one of the disappointments. On a number of occasions, I'd make arrangements to have someone come in to stay with her while I was gone. I still wanted to participate in those activities."[198]

Fred said how he learned it was important to have someone stay with Mary to keep her from wandering or exiting.[199] "Part of my system was…we had a clock that gave the day of the week, the month and the day and the number. We had a calendar that we wrote everything that we did on. And so her routine was to get up, look at the clock to make sure she knew what day, and look at the calendar and know what's going on. And so when I would go someplace, I would always, besides that, write her a note that I went someplace and what time I'd be back. Well, the day that I was 15 minutes late and I came home and she wasn't in the house—so, I did a search. I'd already learned that timing is very important so I didn't wait and I called 911 right away…We live about three miles away. They found her at Publix (grocery store), which is right over here beyond the church. At that time when I said, 'Why did you leave home?' 'Because you said you would be home and you didn't come home—so, I went looking for you.' Oh, that's the most gut wrenching episode!…I mean it just—You just don't know where they are, what's happening. You know they could get in trouble, and it's really tough. After that happened and talking to the sheriffs, I got the something-track, safe-track, care-track[200]…device you wear, that they can locate."[201]

Soon thereafter, Fred was glad he had insisted Mary wear her tracking device. "I came home and she wasn't in the house. Fortunately, she only walked a short way and someone saw her—they saw the bracelet—they called the police. So, when I called the police, they already knew where she was."[202] Sadly, Fred found that even Mary's location device did not prevent her from exiting their house. "She got out one night before we put her in the home. She went next door. This was at nighttime. How she got out without me knowing it, I don't know. She called me up and they said, 'Your wife's over here,' and she was in her nightgown, no shoes or anything. I said, 'I'll be right over to pick her up.' I went over there and picked her up…no trouble coming home, nice and peaceful."[203]

The wandering or exiting behaviors Mary exhibited were also identified by the study's industry professionals as common challenges for caregivers and a tremendous risk for individuals with Alzheimer's or dementia.[204] Often, this is the issue that compels some families to place their loved one into a facility with a secured memory unit.

* * *

Being a second wife in an unsupportive family dynamic, with a husband who would someday be incapable of affirming his wishes, Janice made sure they put all of their legal affairs in order early. "We found a wonderful attorney…a wonderful woman. We went there… You know I never wanted his money. I never wanted to influence the family. I tried to rise above all that…Anyway…when she interviewed us, she could see that he was still very capable of making some decisions"[205]…"and we did the wills and all that. He was cognizant at the time and the attorney established that, that he was doing this in good faith and everything. He got to a point he didn't even want to hear about any of the others. It was not interesting to him. He knew I was taking care of it and that was the last thing he would have done anyway, you know what I mean? He didn't care about that anymore."[206]

"Once I was able to free myself from my own concerns legally, we did a good job."[207]

While George may have initially been less interested, he eventually became more detached in other ways. Janice said that was when his independent mind-set and erratic behaviors grew more problematic. "He would back out the driveway and not even look. It was a good thing we lived at the end of a cul-de-sac, but he almost ran over some people who were walking. He drove—there was never a brake on the car. Just all you did was step on it and go faster and faster and faster."[208] "He got a ticket going up the wrong way, and when he went through a red light, the policeman stopped him. Didn't give him a ticket, but gave him a warning, and it was after that, that he went up the one way and got a ticket. I said, 'That's a waste of a 160 bucks.' I said, 'You've been doing these type of things. I'm not going to be in the car with you anymore. If we're together, I'm going to drive'…It was shortly after that, that I did stop him from driving. I said, 'You're not going to drive,' and I sold both cars, and just bought one in my name."[209]

"Living with him was more like living with a kindergartener… He forgot about this—he forgot about that—and he forgot to clean up his towels and laundry afterwards in the bathroom, so my work was…a lot more."[210] At first, Janice was bothered by his increasing forgetfulness. "He couldn't find a fork that he liked or something. 'What did you do with my fork?' 'Well, it's probably in the drawer.' He had the whole drawer out and everything on the counter looking. Well, and he'd hide things—not hide them, put things away. I'd be looking for them for days and days and days. All of a sudden, he'd say, 'Where are they?' I'd say, 'George, I haven't had a chance to look for them,' when I finally realized how to handle it. At first, I was arguing, 'I didn't touch them!' and 'It wasn't mine!' I mean there were many, many arguments. I would say, 'We'll look for it later.' 'Well, I need it now.' 'Okay, why don't you go watch TV and I'll look for it.' Well, two or three days later it shows up on his table right beside his chair. Now where was it? I have no idea. Absolutely no idea. I still am finding things packed in the corners, underneath in a chair, in back of the TV that we've been looking for, for four or five years. I'm like, 'Okay. Now I understand what's going on.'"[211]

"It was a lot of adjusting on my part, and one of our ladies in our support group, she's so funny, she said, 'Just put that information in the back of your head. It may or may not come up in your situation, but if it does, you won't think, "Oh my gosh, I've got to run to the doctor because this thing is happening."' Okay. I've heard of this before…where they might put on three shirts, or put their shirt on backwards, or put their pants on backwards, or not be able to tie their shoes. Well, I got him Velcro anyway. Make your life easy if you can. So, the support groups, and the time that I had with him, gave me time to adjust my mind. So, yeah. I think it helped. Plus…we were able to do some traveling. I treasure those times that we had."[212]

Adapting to George's reality wasn't easy for Janice, but she said she got better at it over time. "When he got more into it, he got more frustrated and lashed—not lashed out, hitting or anything like that—he did a couple times. He tried to, but his frustration changed his personality a lot. I mean, he would be slamming doors, but he didn't realize that it was because he was forgetful at that point. He'd just think—I don't know what he thought. When he started with the slamming the doors, or 'I'm just gonna go home!' or 'I'm gonna get a divorce!' which he brought up a lot. 'How long have you lived in this house?' Well, in the beginning, I'd tell him, 'Well, we've lived here for years.' Then, I'd go to support group and realize, you don't tell him that. You just say, 'Well, it's a nice house,' or change the subject—or he would pack up: Put one slipper in a bag, his toothbrush, something, and he's 'going home' or 'going to work,' and I would just say to him, 'That's okay, but you know what? You haven't had breakfast yet. How about you sit down—I'll make you some breakfast?' And I'd give him something to eat, turn on the TV, and he'd forget."[213] "Then one night he woke me up at 3:00 in the morning. 'You've got to do something about these people.' I said, 'Excuse?' He said, 'Well, all these people in the living room. Where are they going to sleep? How are you going to help—what can we do?' I said, 'Well, they'll be leaving soon.' I'm sure he said, 'But they're very noisy.' I said, 'Well, why don't you just go back and sit in your chair and relax and take a nap. Hopefully when you wake up, they will have gone.' Of course, he didn't even remember that they were there."[214]

Janice never gave much thought as to where George's delusions may have originated, but she recalled her delight in solving one of those mysteries. "One afternoon, I was sitting there. He says, 'I've got to go out.' I said, 'Where you going?' He said, 'Well, I got to go find my BB gun.' 'Okay, I don't know anything about a BB gun.' He said, 'You wouldn't.' He went out in the back yard, and he's looking around. Next thing I know, he's trying to get in the back door, and I had locked the back door. I had double locked it, so I couldn't even open it. The next door neighbor…she's a nurse, and he's a fireman so they've dealt with this before. They said, 'Gee George, what's the matter?' 'Well, my wife locked me out.' He said, 'Well, why don't we go around to the front door?' 'We have a front door. Yeah, let's go.' Came in the house fine. Finally, his sister was over and I was telling her the story, and she said, 'You know how that happened? At the age about 10, Dad bought him a BB gun. We had a pond out in the back of where he lived. He used to let him go out and shoot the BB's into the pond.' Well, one time his sister went out. Of course, she says, 'I'm being the little brat I always was. I was teasing him, and he miss-shot. He hit the garage, then the BB hit me…from the garage ricochet. Naturally, I run in and tell Dad that George shot me with his BB gun—which he didn't do.' That's where that came from. He evidently went back to that time when his dad—Had I not known that, it just disappeared. It was never mentioned again."[215]

She was still smiling at uncovering the BB gun mystery when she said George did a lot of roaming around the house—especially at night. "It was 12:00. He came in looking for slippers. At 1:30 came in looking for his shoes. Then about 2:30/3:00, he couldn't find his handkerchief. Then the next time couldn't find the bathroom. I mean, it went on all night long. I take him back, and I say, 'The bathroom is right next to your room.' 'No, it isn't.' I said, 'Well, let's take a walk'—after I'd gone to Christine's and I realized how to handle it. Before, I'd argue and we'd have a big to do and he'd get very angry. I take him back. I'd say, 'That's your chair and you were sitting there.' I said, 'And look right here. What's that?' 'That's not my bathroom.' I said, 'Okay. Well, let's go down the hall'…back again and, 'Oh, yeah, that's my bathroom.' Then…another night he comes in looking for the steering wheel of the car. 'Okay, what do I do now?' It's a constant battle…Anyway, I said, 'Look, let's go to the window. Look out the window,' I said, 'Isn't that the car?' He said, 'It certainly is.' 'Don't you suppose the steering wheel's in the car?' Off he goes to sleep. Now, I'm like this. This was constant. You know. There was no sleep. I was afraid to go to sleep."[216]

Supportive neighbors were important for Janice, as George did not confine his roaming to the house when he wandered. "Don't forget now, we moved into a new neighborhood, so I didn't know our neighbors. We—while he was still able to walk—we would get invited to some of the parties. We would go. I didn't hide from anybody what he had, but people were afraid of us I think. They didn't know me. They didn't know this man who definitely had odd behaviors. You know…I had to get him a wanderer's necklace, because he did wander. I almost lost him four times. Even knowing about this wandering condition and thinking that you're smart and intelligent and taking all precautions, he would still get away from me. Oh, it was so maddening."[217]

"One night, we got invited into downtown Tampa. My friend was managing a performing arts theatre. They were having this opening. Now, I have me, my friend, my two neighbors, and I tell them, 'Look, there are a lot of people there.' I said, 'Look, we need to keep an eye on him.' I said, 'You cannot turn your back on this man, because he will try to escape.' Sure enough, I turn around, and he is gone. I start yelling. I said, 'Debbie, you go to the first floor!' That was the floor to get out. 'Lynn, you go to this floor, and Lisa, you go here!' We each took a floor. Well, I ended up running outside, and there he was a good three blocks…I could see him, thank God, heading right towards the Hillsborough River, but I found him. This time, I had some training…I catch up to him. I turn him around, and I have a big smile on my face. If you start screaming at him, he can't react to that in a positive way. He'll just pull away from you. If you smile at him, he'll smile back. He's completely yours. I said, 'Honey, come on, let's go back this way.'"[218]

"I used to think I could leave him in the car. I went shopping. I had to go to Target to get something. I left him in the car. I come out—he's not in the car! Oh, God! I had to go back in the store. I'm running down all the aisles, back and forth, trying to find him. I don't see him. Then, I see this guy running from the back of the store towards the front of the store. He's saying, 'Call 9-1-1! Call 9-1-1!' I said, 'Wait a minute, wait a minute!' I said, 'I'm looking for my husband.' I went. They brought me to him. He was in the warehouse. He was in the back of the store, and he had a shopping cart. He was pushing up the ramp where they deliver things in on this ramp. He was banging and banging, trying to get out. Oh, I was so frightened. I was so scared. I just went over to him. I said, 'Here I am, here I am.' We went home. After that, obviously, I couldn't leave him alone."[219]

"I did give neighbors notes and said, 'If you see him alone, without me, please either call me, or walk with him and kind of direct him home'…After that, when he'd go for walks, I would let him go about four or five houses ahead of me, and I would follow him with a nice cold bottle of water. I'd let him walk. I'd let him walk because I thought it's good for him, and I'd stay a corner behind him, and then when I knew it was getting hot, I'd pull up and I'd just say, 'Hey, you want a ride? I'm going out to eat' or 'Going for an ice cream' or whatever. He'd know it was me. He knew it was me. I kept him home a long time."[220]

* * *

Alice reverted her thoughts back to before the sibling discussions about Mom centered on nursing home or secured memory care unit costs. Early on, most of the family treated Audrey's move into assisted living like she was just giving up a larger house for a cozy apartment so she could stay safe and still have some independence. "The original plan was—'Let Mother stay in the apartment in the ALF as long as possible,' and then when it was needed, we'd probably have to transition her into memory care."[221] To help Audrey make the adjustment from her house to an apartment, Alice spent time online learning how to best help someone with a memory challenge move into new surroundings. On the weekend of the official move, her daughters had their grandmother come visit and spend the night with them at Alice's house. Meanwhile, she and Bill rented a cargo van and spent several hours carefully shuttling Audrey's belongings. "So, before Mom showed up at the ALF, her entire bedroom and her bathroom were decorated with her stuff from her house…Someone needs to feel, when they wake up in the middle of the night and they look around, 'Yeah, it's my house.'"[222]

Silently, I wondered if Alice's siblings had known anything about the two of them working through the night at the assisted living facility, painstakingly recreating Audrey's home environment? I presumed not, since she had already told me that while she was caregiving, she kept most things to herself. Alice seemed to confirm my reasoning with her next statement on the difference between her siblings' perception of Audrey and her own. "I think my concern was they didn't realize it was happening as fast—I think they still thought 'she's going to be Mom for many years' and since I lived near her on a more daily basis, 'she's not going to be Mom for years and years to come. There's less every day. There's less of the mom we remember.'"[223]

Alice had voiced a common frustration of local caregivers. I remembered what one of the study's industry professionals had decided after many years of working directly with dementia patients and their caregivers. "I think that families that are not involved in direct care need to remember the amount of responsibility that goes into providing that care. Not everyone is suited to be a family caregiver, and it can be okay not to be involved, but the reality of knowing, and understanding, and finding ways to support that person who is being the caregiver should be much more relevant than I think often it is."[224]

Alice said Audrey had still wanted to spend time with her other children and then explained how that lead her siblings to believe she was overstating their mother's problems. "Before she went on those trips, she'd often just literally do nothing for a week ahead of time so she had the energy to try to keep up with them. So I think that might be part of it too. She intensely wanted to be normal around them or not affected, and she was able to get away with it for a while. Where she'd come back home and for like a week they'd just be feeding her in her room and you know, basically, she'd just stay in that recliner and not even go to bed. She'd just stay in her recliner for like a week and a half straight because once she came back from that trip, she was just so physically exhausted from trying to be her old self."[225]

Alice paused, with a look of sorrow, before saying, "And that's where part of the resentment grows, from them not seeing it…and them not taking the time to come and see it. 'You guys flew out once a year, came and spent a long weekend with Mom,' but they didn't (see it)."[226] As her sorrowful eyes lingered and her voice trailed off—I thought again of that industry professional's words, "I think denial is a beautiful thing and family members that are not directly involved often don't understand or have a clear picture of what is truly involved in caring for that loved one."[227]

Alice then admitted her mother had always been so good at covering, especially before the diagnosis, that she herself had been guilty of not seeing her mother's quirks as mental failings. Alice straightened her posture, and once again spoke more directly to me as she detailed the saga of her mother's driving issues. "My daughters were over there one time, and my mom drove them. My daughters came to me and said, 'Mom, she can't drive anymore. Don't let your mother drive anymore.' I said, 'Why?' They said, 'Well, she's all over the road.' I said, 'Well, she's done that pretty much her entire life. I don't know that that's necessarily new.'"[228]

Her first driving comment triggered an even earlier memory. "She went to the airport to drop a neighbor off and she couldn't find her way back home and she's like, 'Oh, it's the construction,' and looking back…'No, it wasn't the construction.'"[229] Alice finally realized that risks of denying her mother's driving problems were too dangerous to ignore. "She took my younger daughter and she came back and she said, 'Grandma was driving on the wrong side of the road!'…She didn't have an accident. I think it was she was having problems with her vision and we finally told her it's time to give up the car. It's just time to give up the car and she wasn't really happy."[230]

However, Alice voiced an uncomfortable difference between telling a parent not to drive and actually getting them to stop driving. "It's very hard to take the keys away from someone who still feels like they're mostly fine…We were finally able to completely take the keys away from her. We probably had that go on longer than it should have, but it was very challenging to make that work."[231] She and her husband finally told Audrey, "'Your doctor said you can't drive.' Dr. Sweeney had…a way that she seemed to understand. She said, 'Audrey, if you drive now that I've diagnosed you with dementia and you hurt someone, they're going to come back after me and say, 'Why'd you let her drive?' So, I can't let you drive anymore.' So, Mom kind of understood that. 'I can't drive because it'll get the doctors in trouble,' and she seemed to be okay with that."[232]

Regardless of the effort it took to get Audrey to stop driving, Alice was relieved, knowing it meant her mother would be safer. What came next concerned even her brother. During one of Audrey's family visit trips, "She walked down the street and came back and she tried to get into the neighbor's house. Granted, it looked similar to my brother's house, but it wasn't my brother's house and it was enough dissimilar that she should have known. The police were called because she was trying to get into the next-door-neighbor's house, and she was trying to get in, and they didn't know. Some stranger was trying to get in, they didn't know who it was, and then they called police, and…they were just about as kind as they could be…They were just as kind as they could be, and they said, 'You know, you just need to be watching really closely if this becomes more frequent.'"[233]

* * *

Yvonne glanced at the smaller portrait frame, which held a picture of Richard in his military uniform alongside her grandmother. She looked down at the other loose photos on the table and smiled at a picture of him in a convertible car. "He would get very upset about not being able to drive. They have men's luncheons where I live where the old elderly men would go out to lunch a couple of times a month and things like that. He would drive sometimes, so he went out with Keith. Keith's passed away too now, but he was a wonderful man. Him and Keith went out to lunch, and they ended up going all the way up the highway in the wrong direction—two hours! Keith kept trying to get my grandfather to turn around. He could be kind of stubborn…Eventually they show up and Keith comes up to me and says, 'Yvonne, I think it might be time. I know this is difficult, but maybe it's time for him not to be driving anymore.' What I had to do to solve that problem, because he would get very angry with me. 'Who was I to tell him not to drive?' I had Dr. Townsend write out on a prescription pad that the doctor's orders were that 'Richard should not be driving anymore.' He respected his doctor. He took his word and he would follow his doctor's orders, so I was able to use that in moments when he was adamant, like, 'I need to drive! Go get me the keys—you can't tell me what to do and not drive!' 'That's not me, Grandpa. I'm not the one telling you. See, your doctor said.' It worked with him."[234]

She suddenly smiled brightly to tell me of one memorable drive Richard wanted to take her on. "One time, we were out walking the dogs, and he said to me, 'Go get my car keys—we're going to Europe!' Now, I hadn't gone to caregiver's support group. I had read a few articles on Alzheimer's. I was just being introduced on how to handle situations as a caregiver, so I was still in the mode of reasoning with him. He was brilliant. He was an archeologist—he was a very intelligent man. I was trying to reason with him, 'No, Grandpa, we can't drive to Europe.' I'm trying to explain, there's this big ocean between us…so I was thinking…'I will go get this map and I will show him on the map that there's the Atlantic Ocean between us and Europe so we can't.' It didn't work, because he couldn't. He was broken. To try to reason with someone with Alzheimer's doesn't work. I started learning those things, but I hadn't at that point. Here I am, the granddaughter, trying to tell my grandfather he can't do what he wants to do, and this is the man who raised me. He's like, 'Go get the keys—let's get in the car!' I prayed a lot through my time as a caregiver. I remember standing there going, 'Lord, how do I help him? What do we do here?' What came to my mind was, 'He's a very old-fashioned gentleman, so he wouldn't like to show up unannounced at somebody's house.' I said, 'Grandpa, we can't go now—they're not expecting us.' Just that, 'They're not expecting us.' He was like, 'Oh, okay. That would be rude.' I learned to enter into where he was, into his world."[235]

She thought it was funny that her grandfather thought someone showing up unexpectedly was wrong, yet when she was still working—she had to worry about him answering the door. "He'd answer the door for anybody. I'd preached over and over and over again, 'Don't let anybody in the house that you don't know. Do not give out any information, no phone numbers, no nothing.'"[236] Eventually, Richard was confused by some of the people Yvonne had come into the house to help, but she said the dogs were always a calming presence for him. "He talked to them like they were normal people—didn't understand why they didn't understand him when he was talking to them. 'They should understand this and know that,' and…I'm like, 'Well, no, they're just animals. They're smart…the dogs are smart, but they're not that smart,' and I joked with him…He'd sit there and he'd be talking to the dog and I'm going, 'Grandpa,' I said, 'You're gonna make me rich if that dog talks to me one day or talks back to you one day,' and he'd laugh."[237]

Whether it was driving to Europe or talking to the dogs, Yvonne felt if it made sense to him, it was up to her to find some way to connect and redirect. "I realized that you cannot really argue at all with him, or try and correct him in any way, shape, or form. Best just to agree with him. That's what I always did. Just agree and maybe change the subject, or if it was like going to the doctor, or whatever, to always be, 'Hey, we're going to go eat lunch. Don't you want McDonald's?' I'd throw lunch out there, because he loved to go out and eat, so I kind of focused on things that I knew he'd like to do, to get him to do things that I knew he wouldn't agree to do, and it worked."[238]

Yvonne looked up from the photo collection, leaned back in her chair to say, "I think I was really blessed. My grandfather was really blessed in that aspect, because he wasn't angry a lot. He wasn't combative. He actually had a lot more peace during his time of

Alzheimer's than he did as I remember him growing up. He was actually very angry without the Alzheimer's. It's kind of interesting. He had a lot more peace later in the progression of that."[239]

She began to rearrange the photos on the table and stacked the convertible picture on top of two others. Before Richard's friend, Keith, had been unable to get him to turn the car around, Yvonne said the first time he got lost driving was really odd. "He went to go to the grocery store. My friend's father…was the fire chief…somebody that worked for him actually found Grandpa like six counties away from where we lived, nowhere near in the same direction that he was supposed to be going, and he was completely clueless that he was even lost! He stopped at the firehouse because he wanted to buy a hoagie. The house that we grew up in was right behind the firehouse, and every Wednesday they would sell dollar hoagies. He saw a firehouse, and he went in and asked them about buying a hoagie. That's how they ended up finding him."[240]

Once he stopped driving, Yvonne still worried about him getting lost. "A couple of times, he would take the dogs out for a walk and get lost. 'Oh, where's Grandpa?' I'd go out and I'd look for him. The neighborhood is very nice. The neighbors all knew him, so they would bring him home. Sometimes he would take the dogs out for a walk and he'd get to a different building, and he'd just decide to sit there for a real good long time. That was a little scary, thinking maybe he had wandered away and not knowing where he was." Her brows lifted and her eyes widened as she continued her thought, "Just scared that he would get hurt…We live at *Westfield Palms*, so it is sort of gated. I didn't know if he would get confused and wander out beyond there. I prayed, and then I walked around and looked for him. I did find him. That was when he was sitting on the bench, and then other times neighbors would bring him back. It probably happened maybe ten times or something like that."[241]

It wasn't only the neighbors watching out for her grandfather that made Yvonne thankful during those challenging years. "One time, we were at a restaurant, and it was just the right kindness at the right time. It was in a very difficult week. I took him out to eat, and we're having a conversation. He was very repetitive with, 'Where is my wife? Did she run off with another man?' Like, 'No, Grandpa, she loved you. You were married for 60 years. Nanny didn't go have an affair.' We were in the middle of that cycle. I went to go pay the bill…the lady at the counter says, 'Don't worry about it, Honey. The people next to you took care of your bill.' I mean, it still brings tears to my eyes, because it was just that little kindness, in a moment of just struggle, that somebody had observed. Just a little kindness goes a long way."[242]

Limits

Fred tried to simply incorporate Mary's reality into their daily life. "If she said she went here last night or 'I was playing cards in Tampa' or whatever—you go, 'Oh, well that was good. Did you win any money?' I mean, you just gotta go…They call it a 'medical fib.'"[243, 244] He gave another example. "'I went down and saw my mother. She's in a nursing home.' I said, 'Oh yeah, that's right.' Well her mother died 15 years ago, but she went down to see her mother and she did this or that. So, her long-term memory is not good, but it's still 'sputtering,' I guess is the word."[245]

For a while, Mary's slipping into her own reality did not stop him from taking care of her at home, but it did complicate things. "Sometimes it was difficult getting her doctor's appointments, because no matter what time it was, it took forever to get her dressed. Get her dressed. I'd go in the bathroom for two minutes and she'd either be undressed, or putting other clothes over the others."[246]

As her mind grew worse, even driving became more compli-cated. Once, Fred got Mary strapped into the front passenger seat. He opened up the driver's door and he said she shouted, "'You can't drive this van!' 'Why not?' 'My husband will kill me! He doesn't let anybody drive his van!'"[247]

Fred said Mary often forgot who he was, but wouldn't ask who he was. "She'd say, 'My daughter wants to talk to you.' So, I'd pick up the phone and she would say, 'Dad, she wants to know who this strange man is sitting out in the patio. She doesn't know how to get rid of him.'"[248]

His daughter wasn't always successful in calming Mary down when she forgot who Fred was—like the time he was rushing to change her insulin pump. "One morning before support group, it's time to change it. Take everything off. Everything's all set. I got all the insulin in the pump. Go to put it on, 'What are you doing?' 'I got to put the site in you so you can have your insulin.' 'Well, I don't know who you are. I don't know that you know what you're doing. You're not going to put that into me!' I'd said to myself, 'I got to be able to take care of her. If I can't take care of her, I'll have to place her.' I said, 'Mary, I'm your husband. I'm Fred.' 'Well, I don't know…' I called up my daughter—she talked to my wife, and I said, 'Talk to Mom, and tell her who I am.' It took about an hour and a half before I could finally…I finally got it in, but I said, 'You know, if I can't take care of her medical needs, if she doesn't trust me, I have to do something.'"[249]

He said he doesn't really expect her to recognize him anymore. Fred forced a smile to say, "I don't think she has any clue as to what our relationship is except that I'm that guy that comes in. One of my friends up there says, 'That cute guy that comes in every day.'"[250]

His smile gave way as he talked about his concern for how frightening things must seem to her when she's in a confused state of mind. "Sometimes she'd feel bugs crawling on her,"[251] adding, "She's hit me several times, when the dementia took—when she gets totally confused, didn't know who I was. She couldn't hurt me…she was just mad, confused."[252]

Still mired in his concern for her scared perspective, he admitted there was a period when she did actually frighten him. "A couple weeks, she didn't even recognize me when we went to bed. She said, 'You're not my husband!' I found about eight knives—steak knives—underneath the mattress!…At that time, I knew there was something wrong as far as her brain was concerned. I worked through it, and I got out the marriage license, the whole wedding thing, showing pictures and things like that. Then, we was able to go to sleep that night, no problems. There was times I'd be on the couch, and every sound that was made, I'd wake up. You would too, if somebody had knives in the bed!"[253]

It wasn't only Mary's confusion Fred had to deal with. "Over the next year or two, there was a very steady but very gradual decrease in her abilities…It eventually got to the point where I had to shower her."[254] "We kind of joke in the support group too, that if we had taken as many showers when we were younger, together, our daughter would have had siblings. You learn how to do it and I thought I was doing a pretty good job—and I think I was doing a pretty good job. It just got to be a little overwhelming toward the end. The 24/7 aspect of it, just wore me down."[255] Fred found someone to assist Mary with "bathing twice a week, so I supplemented in between. As she progressed, she became incontinent,"[256] which he said was the most "significant" change in her progression. "First it was just urinary and then subsequently it was also fecal. I was surprised because in my own mind, I kind of thought that that was going to be my line in the sand. I was very surprised at how adaptable the human animal can become under the most extraordinary circumstances."[257] "They recommended disposal diapers, or pants, whatever it is. I was resistant to that for a while because during the day she will go to the—when she was awake, she would go to the bathroom. She didn't have as much time when she realized she had to go—but she would go. It was the night time that was the problem. By wearing these disposal ones…the advantage of it—it whips the moisture away from the body so they're not going to get sore from the urination. Once I accepted that and let her wear them, that made life a lot easier too."[258] "We went along and, again from the support group, I had all the information I needed so far as Depends, mattress pads and all that kind of thing. I was taking advantage of the knowledge of those that had gone before us."[259]

Even with peer advice, the strain of Mary's decline took its toll on Fred. "My initial thought was, 'Okay, we got a plan, we'll execute it, and everything will be fine.' As things degraded with her abilities, then I said, 'This doesn't always work'…I admit I was one who waited too long to get help…it put too much of a burden on us. It started affecting our health. I said I don't want to go through that because… 'If you're gonna be a caregiver, you gotta be healthy.'"[260] Fred prioritized Mary's care ahead of everything else. "I just let the house go. It needs…Well, we moved in 14 years ago—I haven't painted since. I'd hire somebody to mow the lawn, or fertilize it, but there's a lot of…We've paid somebody to trim—we have six humongous oak trees. There's always something to do around the house. I had an old pickup truck that I wanted to fix up, and I gave that away."[261]

Princess stood up to stretch, making Fred pause for a moment. When she'd settled herself back down, he looked up and told me about Mary's final year at home with them. "During the summer and early fall, it was like she fell off a cliff. She started losing her mobility. She started losing her verbalization. She started losing her ability to feed herself."[262] Stability concerns became a factor in Fred's reluctant placement of Mary. "I believe, in talking to the nurses, she has many years to live yet—even though she's been in it for years…so, I'm not fearful of her dying. But I'm fearful if I were to leave her alone, she would do something that could get hurt. She's fallen a couple of times."[263] "She'd pretty much be able to walk in the house with a little bit of assistance—there was enough walls, enough stuff for her to…

One time, she slipped off the toilet in the bathroom. She'd fallen a few times in the house. One time she slipped off the toilet, wedged herself, it's a small bathroom, between the toilet and the door. I could not get her to move. I couldn't open the door more than this much. I called the fire department, and they said, 'Well, is there a window there?' I said, 'Let's just cut the door, that it was a cheap door.' So, I get a buzz saw. I said, 'I got a buzz saw.' Anyhow, I cut the door enough for the firemen…They were trained—they knew how to lift her…One fireman was able to at least move her where they were able to open the door."[264]

Suddenly Fred's voice disappeared, his eyes filled with tears, and neither of us said a word. I quietly moved the box of tissues within his reach and just sat there—letting him take as long as he needed. After 20 to 30 seconds, Fred wiped his eyes and, with his face still covered by his hand, began speaking. "I'm sorry. It was the hardest times because it was the most wearing out of me. It was totally wearing me mentally and physically, both I think. I was exhausted…I began having to check her blood pressure before—she's got blood pressure medicines four times a day—I was having to check them before each

time. She was taking eight different pills, or, no I'm sorry, four different pills, but eight times a day, because some of them she was taking
twice a day. They were at all different times throughout the day."[265]
"I was exhausted 24 hours a day. I slept like a dead person. She did
too. She slept very well at night but I really wasn't getting any rest. I
don't know what was going on in my head during those hours. It just
got to the point where I knew I was hurting myself much more than
I was helping her."[266] Fred had emerged from behind the tissue and
his speaking pace was faster. "You have all these months and years, in
most cases, to build up to this. So it's not a surprise when they suddenly get to the point that you can't care for them anymore… It's of
course, it's a shock, but it's not anything that's unexpected. You know
it's going to happen, but you're just not sure when."[267]

Whether it was guilt or just a reprieve from his nonstop caregiving duties for Mary, Fred initially placed her in a facility, then
changed his mind. "I took her out of the home after about 14 days.
I thought, 'I can handle this.' Then, she broke out the back window
and tried to get out the door. I had locks on the doors, because I
didn't want her wandering around. She couldn't get out the door, so
she was arguing with me in the hallway. I picked her up and took her
in the bedroom and closed the door. Within two minutes, she had the
back window broke out, and she threatened to break the television
before, by breaking out the window."[268] Fred said he had expected
Mary to be calmer because she was back home. "It finally dawned on
me that something else might have been taking place other than just
the disease. I suspected urinary tract infection. Having been coming
to the support group meetings here since shortly after she had been
diagnosed, I heard a lot about all that kind of thing."[269] "We put her
in the hospital…at the suggestion of the EMTs. The best thing that
ever happened as far as I'm concerned. While she was there, they had
her admitted, cleaned up, taken samples, urine and so on and her
diagnosed with the UTI within about two, two and a half hours of
hitting the front door. I think she went in on a Tuesday and she was
discharged on Saturday. In the meantime, I made arrangements to

have her go to a health and rehab center, skilled nursing center. She's been there ever since."[270]

* * *

Janice looked past me to the corner of the small conference room as she paused to prepare herself for what she would say next. "I remember telling my leader, 'The saddest day for me will be the day that he doesn't recognize me,' and of course that day came, and I realized in being in the support group, that he didn't recognize me because he was diverted back…and he was looking for his 40-year-old wife who had long brown hair and a lot thinner body—which was not me. So, most of the time, he knew me, but there were several times when he didn't know who I was, and that's sad. That's sad."[271]

Still staring into space, she told of George's general decline. "I mean, gradually, it seemed like, gradually he lost interest in all the things that he liked. Like reading, he stopped reading. He was an avid reader and he just stopped reading and I mean, it's because he couldn't read. Didn't understand the words anymore…I mean, I noticed one thing…his world became so limited and I thought that was sad. He had me and that's really the only place he felt truly comfortable. Everything I did, I did with him. It was—We were able to do dinner with people if they could—but, even that, I began to feel uncomfortable with having people over because it's not easy. Most people don't know how to deal with somebody with Alzheimer's and you got somebody that's constantly repeating what they're saying and…I mean he would do really weird stuff. I remember one time he went to the bathroom and our guest came out and said, 'I think he had an accident.' It was all over the place, you know what I mean? It was a mess in there. I didn't want to expose people to that."[272]

Janice turned back toward me. "The interesting part about caregiving is that when you're in the midst of it, you don't look for reasons why you do what you do. You just do what you do and for me, I became so embroiled in the pragmatic or practical matters of caregiving that I often lost sight of the reason that you do these things. You know that you're doing this because you love him, or you do it because it's the right thing to do. I don't know. You do it because you want to feel good about yourself at the end of the journey. Those things never—I don't know. They didn't weigh on my mind a lot. I just went into action."[273] "He didn't need a shower every day but I insisted on showering every day. Well, he hated that. He got to the point that the people that came in wouldn't even bother trying. So, I'm having to get him into the shower, hose him down basically, and I just figured out something too because they came and they put in a special thing where you can spray and a chair and a handrail. The chair, I kept in there, but he thought the chair was the toilet, so here I'd clean him up—and I'd get him to go to the bathroom first so he'd be all nice and clean afterwards—and he would go right there on the toilet—so then, that was the cleaning thing. The cleaning issue became a problem. The toileting became a real problem. Pretty much, I kept him to the end though."[274]

She seemed glad that she did most of George's caregiving without hiring everyday home health aides. "I didn't want them in my house. I'm a very private person and I don't do anything wrong here, but it's my house. I don't want people wandering around—that kind of people—I don't mean family or friends. I don't care about that. But, I didn't like having these people here. I wasn't real impressed with the help that I got so—nobody could be as—nobody can love your loved one like you can love them."[275] "Because he had that 'sundowner thing' that later in the day, he got worse…by 3:00, it was okay, I could work around that. Then, it got to be just too difficult to do and too much for me to handle. So, I did have somebody come in twice a week. The sending him out anywhere just didn't work very well."[276]

"Half the people would say, 'You should put him away.' You know, 'Now is time.'"[277] Janice said she was too busy to hear them. "Get up, two and a half, three hours to get him a shower, but it's like post-traumatic stress syndrome. I mean, you just do it, and it's hard, and you don't know it until they are placed—that your life has been so difficult—and that you didn't have a life, and you did not know it at the time…You go from social groups being smaller to almost nothing unless it's your support group, because people do not understand that do not live with this disease."[278] "There's so many things that you have no concept. Every day was a different day. No two days were the same."[279]

Her words trailed off, ahead of Janice sharing his ultimate departure from the home. "At the end, I remember one day we were just sitting…and he was holding the dog, which he loved. Our dog was his company. He was holding the collar but he was hurting the dog and I was trying to get him so he'd let the dog go and he said, 'I'm going to butcher you!' And, he's a big man. He's scary. If he decided he was going to hurt me, he could do it very easily. He could kill me in a heartbeat. That's when I decided, I can't deal with this. I just couldn't do it."[280] "He picked up the dog and threw her. I thought, 'Don't touch my dog! Don't hurt my dog!'…I knew not to confront him, but…I stood up, and I was in his face, and I said, 'What did you do?' And he, at that point, pulled his fist back, and he says, 'I'll kill you!' and I said, 'George, it's me! It's me! It's me!' and he swung his fist out. I put my hand in front. I thought he broke my finger. Hit my hand. I jumped…I grabbed my shoes, grabbed my purse. I knew where my keys were—I took her, and I went and got out of the house—and the police did come…I called the police. I said, 'This is not domestic violence, this is dementia'—and the police came. I gave him Lorazepam…By the time they came, he was back in bed asleep. He was fine, but I told hospice, 'I need him gone. I need him gone,' and it's a very strange feeling when you know that they will never come back in the house again. The slippers are there, the cup of coffee's there, whatever. It's very final, even though I knew he was still alive, and I didn't know if he'd live another year or two."[281]

Sometimes Janice brought the dog when she went to visit George in the facility. "I'd take her in the room and she'd lick his face all over. And then she sat down in front of him and they were just happy…If I took her, it was like we were all together again at home." She smiled again. "He'd call me, 'The love of his life.' I'd say, 'What's my name?' 'The love of my life'…And he was kind. He used to be an abrasive businessman, and now he was really sweet—so it was easier."[282] She laughed that she wasn't the only woman there who thought George was sweet. "One lady put him to bed and covered him up and kissed him goodnight. One sat out in the hall and waited for me to leave."[283] Still smiling, she said she knew the residents were harmless.

"Every night, when I left the facility, I went to their machine and I put some music on…I liked to do little studies myself, and I watched them migrate to the TV and they'd sit down, and they'd calm down.[284] But nobody turned that on… They didn't have time because they were short staffed…The other thing is, people just disappear. Like about 8:00, I couldn't find anybody. Somebody should've been available, and somebody should've been held accountable."[285] "I mean, these people, it's a hard job. I don't think they get paid enough, but they were not going to love my husband, and so I didn't want to leave him with people that didn't love him. Just treated him like an object…The home I put him in—I remember, when I would go to visit him, he would be like this—all hunched over, like he'd been punished. I asked him, and I really couldn't get an answer from him, but it was basically—I think they were making fun of him or they weren't being nice to him, nice enough."[286] "I saw probably 65% of the people without anyone…You know that they were not as clean… I'd said, 'George is not gonna get better. I know that, and he's gonna get worse, but you're gonna take care of him. It's very expensive here and if I pay for this, you have to do it.' I told the girls that. 'And don't let me come in here at the end and find him on the couch…with feces at the back of his neck.' I said, 'Don't let that happen again! I mean that!' And then I'd take them a box of donuts the next day. You know, I tried to reward them and I told them, 'I know your job's hard. It's very hard.' So they were good to him."[287]

After recalling George's placement, Janice's voice trembled with defeat. "There were times when I wished that he wasn't here. I wished he'd die. Then, I'd feel guilty about that. Then, I thought, 'Oh my God, it's seven years. How much longer can I go?'"[288]

* * *

The appreciative smile Alice wore when she spoke of the police officers' kindness and concern during her mother's wandering incident at her brother's faded quickly. While it had affirmed her belief that Audrey could not function well on her own, it also forecasted she might not be able to stay in the assisted living facility forever. There had not actually been a discussion on a memory care unit with Audrey. "She flat out refused to leave the town she retired to… that was her number one thing that she told me when we signed the papers for everything. She goes, 'I don't ever want to leave my house and I don't ever want to leave this town.' Well, leaving the house at least was her choice when we did it. She knew that she had to go. She didn't want to, but she knew she had to…She was very clear that she did not want to leave town. To that extent, it gave me complete confidence in that I was doing what she wanted…Otherwise, I would have moved her closer to where we were so I could give her more care, but that wasn't an option."[289] Alice slowly shook her head as she continued. "Convincing her that she needed to leave the house was hard, but she was still aware enough of what was going on that it was a—she wasn't emotional about it because again, she was that classic 1960's wife. Right? That 'Everything's great'…The whole world could be crashing down but, 'We're gonna be happy and make everyone think, anyway, we're happy about it.' So, she pulled that off so it wasn't hard for me, but I imagine that was, probably, really difficult for her."[290]

I wondered if Alice had projected her own feelings into the depiction of Audrey's outward calmness, despite suspected emotional distress. She said her mother's acceptance to move into the assisted living facility actually preceded her siblings'. "My sister wasn't as on board, but I said, 'Let's do something about this'—We went and we saw…three ALFs. Then my sister said, 'Look, I have rented a convertible and I'm going to take Mother…and she and I are going to have a day together.' I said, 'That's wonderful.' She and Mother took off for the day and when they got back, my sister was completely on board. I have a feeling, though my sister and I have never discussed it, that one of those incidents happened while she was with my sister, and my sister suddenly realized, 'Whoa, this is exactly as bad as it could be.'"[291]

Audrey's insistence on staying at an assisted living facility near her friends to maintain her social circle, instead of family, did not live up to her expectations. Alice explained, "It's very hard, especially when your friends are in their 80s and have their own problems…In the very beginning, they would take her places, but as it got more difficult, they didn't want to take her places…She couldn't understand why no one would take her…because it's a liability. You have this other person who's 80-some taking an 84-year-old with dementia out, who, as you're walking, doesn't remember. She's looking around at the sites and doesn't realize she needs to look down and step, and she's going to trip, and how to use the walker, and the thinking isn't all there. They didn't want the responsibility. She was mad…I told her, I said, 'Mom, you know, they're all older.' I just made it out that she switched from one of those metal walkers…to the heavier walker with the seat and those were heavier, much, much heavier. To have to lift them and fold them and put them in your trunk, I said, 'A lot of your friends probably don't want to have to do that because…it's too heavy.'"[292] Alice said in spite of her mother's isolation, she had understood Audrey's friends' circumstances. "In the very beginning, that was fine. It's when she got a little bit worse that people didn't feel as comfortable taking her to places…She was incontinent…I think that's when they were all very uneasy and I couldn't blame them."[293]

Alice closed her eyes, seeming to look back at images of her mother—wanting to accurately capture what she had seen change over time. "She was a very strong, educated, verbal person and she became very meek, very quiet, very timid…She was afraid to go anywhere…afraid to do anything. She wouldn't make a decision. It was like she became this terrified child—which was hard to see."[294]

When Alice opened her eyes, they were moist again as she described another image of Audrey that still haunted her. "She started screaming one day—'They give me all these medicines! They come and they clean me! They're cleaning me, but no one is cleaning out my brain! I can't think! I just can't think! They just got to clean out the brain!' She would say that over and over." I handed Alice another tissue as she finished, "She would remember things from her youth and I would try and keep her focused on reminiscing…she did better, 'You see, that part of my brain is clean. They just need to clean out the rest of it.' That's what she—That was hard. That was hard."[295]

Having a full-time job, plus her own family, made it more challenging to watch over Audrey's care—especially with a 45-minute drive to visit. "She knew I came every day. Every time I would get there and say, 'How are you?' She goes, 'I'm good now.' Every day, she knew I was going to be there every day after work and everyone kept telling, 'You got to stop doing that. You got to start going every other day or go every few days.' I just—it's easy to say that to somebody. It's a lot easier to say that than it is if you're living it....I was driving over there all the time and feeling guilty that I was never doing enough."[296]

Alice's nightly visits to her mother's assisted living facility apartment were usually more about chores than just spending time with Audrey. She wanted her mother to be in a cleaner environment than the staff had time to do. Alice said she had become a regular in the facility's laundry room and was constantly bringing in shopping bags to ensure her mother would have enough mattress pads and adult diapers for the aides to change her.

When I asked for more elaboration on her family's thoughts on her daily caregiving efforts, Alice took a long breath and sighed. "They were understanding and knew that I felt the need to go over there all the time, but they were very concerned...They were always afraid I was going to fall asleep driving home. That was their bigger concern, was they were very concerned that I was driving home tired and late...They would start calling me at nine, 'You leaving?' 'Yeah, I'm leaving soon,' but they knew I wasn't. They were not happy with me driving home late and tired...I wasn't taking care of myself. I wasn't sleeping, probably stressed."[297]

As we sat there in Alice's clean and extremely well-organized office, I envisioned her having tried to keep Audrey's apartment just as tidy. She may have noticed my gaze at her obvious penchant for order and told me that she eventually learned to make some compromises. "I did relinquish doing the laundry. The facility finally convinced me, 'Let us do her laundry. We'll just take care of the laundry.' Having to relinquish something was hard...and they were not doing it the way I would do it. If my mother only knew—and she was so meticulous on how her clothes were folded and if I fold it, 'No, fold it with the pleats this way. You button the shirt.' She had one dresser drawer of her printed sweaters and one…for the solids. Oh God, you go to the ALF, the clothes would come back rolled up, stuffed in a drawer…I remember I moved her in and I had a drawer of her little nightgowns, and a drawer of pants, and a drawer of—Oh gosh, no, everything was just rolled up." Shaking her head again, Alice began to smile. "You know, you just have to learn to let that stuff go. It's really not important and I started to notice, 'You know what? Whatever they put on my mother, she didn't even notice any more if she matched, if she didn't match.' That part I let go because it didn't have—effect on her health."[298]

Once Alice had stated learning to delegate chores for her mother was difficult—I asked if delegation had been an accepted option for her at work. "I think the corporate space looks at this and says, 'It's fine that you do that, but you still need to get all your work done.' So, it creates so much extra stress…There's not really flexibility to be able to say, 'We're comfortable with peeling back some of the expectation that we have.' It's full bore all the time."[299] Then, Alice added that she had encountered an entirely different experience from her work environment earlier in her career. "I think when kids are sick—like really sick, like in the hospital kind of sick—there's so much sympathy. My own child spent a month in the ICU after she was born, and there was never any discussion or expectation placed on me of doing work during that time. It was kind of like, 'You tend to your family, and that's most important.'"[300] Upon hearing herself surprisingly still bothered by the vastly different work responses, she stiffened her posture and dialed back her comments on the workplace impact of her mother's care needs. "I mean, at the very end, when I had to take off a lot, luckily where I work was very, very understanding and I had a lot of vacation and sick leaves. That worked out very well… It affected, if anything, my health, just because I was so tired, just too tired, not taking care of myself."[301]

After another glance through the glass office door, Alice pivoted her body and her thoughts. She redirected from how her caregiving challenged her work to how work had challenged her caregiving. "One particular evening, I was actually on the other side of Florida for a business meeting…my phone rings. It is the ALF. Mother has come down out of her room, and this is very, very late before she became needing 24-hour care…Anyway, she evidently had been in her room, looked around, and decided that this was not her home in Atlanta and that she needed to go home. She left her apartment, evidently knew enough to get on the elevator—there was no elevator at her Atlanta home—went down the four floors to the lobby, and tried to get somebody to help her go home from there. Now, I was… four hours away and Mother phoned. Actually, the ALF phoned me. I talked to the ALF, I talked to Mother to try to help calm her down, and I did manage to calm her down on the phone, but we had to deal with the idea of where this was going, and it was a bit of a strain because I was four hours away. Best I could have done was pack up from where I was, throw everything in the car, head four hours over there and deal with Mom face-to-face. Luckily…with my help, we calmed her down, we got her back into the room and she actually stayed. I was very, very concerned that I was going to be getting a call within the next hour that she was out of the room again, but it didn't happen. She went back into the room, took her evening pills, lay down on the bed, went to sleep, so I was very fortunate… She didn't even remember that she hadn't remembered. It was one of those incidents."[302]

Other times, Audrey did think the apartment was still her home in Atlanta. Alice recalled, "We were in the apartment at the ALF, at one point, when my sister said she was coming to visit and my mother said, 'I got to go down the hall and fix the guest bedrooms…' There's no hall and there's no guest bedrooms. She was thinking of our original childhood house—800 miles away. Later, my husband and I said, 'An 800-mile hallway, that's a long hall!'"[303]

Alice suddenly slipped back into a quiet, self-conversation— slowly reflecting on Audrey's decline. "I lost Mom about 18 months before Mom passed away. It was okay but difficult to deal with. To have to deal with the day-to-day work of it, plus the emotions, plus all the things every human being has to deal with in their life, difficulties at the office, whatever else, was very difficult, and I think caused the period of those emotional things to be drawn out."[304]

Her mother's growing confusion led Alice to make the sad decision to move Audrey from the assisted living facility apartment she had agreed to a few years earlier. "She wasn't able to stay in the assisted living place anymore. She needed too much care, so we moved her over to…a memory care unit."[305] "She did have to go into a lockdown facility because she wandered a lot."[306] Alice said her visits were much different in the memory care unit. Gone were her mother's belongings, the dresser full of wrinkled clothes, and the bright curtains she and Bill had hung in her apartment to remind her of home. She remembered seeing Audrey after she'd been moved out of the assisted living apartment. "We saw her when she was in lockdown, and I said, 'Mom,' I said, 'I'm trying to collect some memories,'… and I said, 'Can you think of anything?' She said, 'Nah,' and I said, 'How about the time you all went to Niagara Falls?' She goes, 'I didn't go to Niagara Falls.'…So we realized at that point…her long-term memory had started to go."[307]

"She always knew who I was. She'd mess up on the names. Right? She'd call me my sister's name sometimes…My hunch is that she didn't really know who I was. Certainly when we moved her into the memory care unit, she didn't know…she lost awareness of that."[308] Alice swallowed hard—she was choked up recalling the memory care visit. She discovered she wasn't the only person Audrey could no longer remember. "She was wandering around…and I remember going up to her and said, 'Mom, it looks like you're looking for something. Can I help you?' 'Yeah.' I said, 'What are you looking for?' She says, 'I'm looking for me. I lost me.' I almost lost it—I didn't know how to respond."[309]

Whatever restraint Alice had mustered during that visit to keep from crying was no longer present. I asked if she wanted to pause the interview. She said no, but we recorded 30 seconds of silence before she shared a final thought on the strain of placing her mother into a lockdown facility. "The biggest heartbreak that I've had…I went to the memory ward with my husband to put my mother in the memory ward…They let my mother follow us to the exit door. My mother said, 'If you all would let me go home with you, I'll be real good.' That broke my—I don't know…my husband is a tough… man… He and I got into the car and we just sat there and cried."[310]

* * *

Speaking on the kindness of strangers continued to make Yvonne smile. "People, they were so kind. I experienced a lot of kindness going out with him and things like that, for sure. We went to the zoo, and he had a scooter—and he nearly ran a lady over!"[311] She laughed, shaking her head. "Yeah…everywhere we went—I can't recall in that six, seven years, one experience of negativity out in the public where somebody observed something and didn't say something kind…If I pulled up somewhere to a restaurant, and I didn't have a friend with me and I was by myself—so, you're in the dilemma of, get the walker out or the wheelchair, whatever…pull up to the restaurant walkway, get him on that safely, go park as quick as you can. I would have people hold the door open, say to me, 'I'll sit here with him while you get the car parked.'"[312]

"I had started taking him to the adult daycare center. Eventually I stopped working, and he had a certain amount of resources that he had put into that could provide for a home health aide to come. It was minimal time. It was probably two hours once a week or something like that, but I would use that time where they would come early in the morning at, say like, 5:00 and I could sleep a little longer. They would dress him and give him his medicine and breakfast and then go. Part of that I used for the adult daycare center. He could socialize and they had crafts and the nurses were on staff there. It's such a wonderful resource, but somebody told me about that, and so I'd meet different people through these things. They would give me more information, pamphlets, reading materials, things like that that really helped me understand, and I probably got more understanding from that than the doctor and the neurologist when I think about it looking back. Because…once I entered that world of caregiving, I sort of met other caregivers."[313]

"I don't regret one moment of it because the context of my family, the way that the relationship was with my grandfather growing up, and the way that it was in his later years, was just completely restoring and beautiful. I had such a great relationship with him and we had fun. It was—he was a different person, not just because of the Alzheimer's, but because he had peace with God later in his life, so that was all part of the picture. I wouldn't change one second of that. It was very hard, very challenging, very demanding, very exhausting, but very rewarding and healing, and beautiful and a lot of really positive things…We went on adventures. I took him to the circus. We went out to the dog park. He didn't sit around. I was like, 'Grandpa took me everywhere, I'm going to take Grandpa everywhere.' It was so beautiful at the circus because he had a moment of clarity, and he looked at me and he said, 'You took me to the circus.' I was like, 'Yeah, Grandpa.' Because I have a really good childhood memory of going to the circus with him, so that's really beautiful."[314] Yvonne had expected Richard to enjoy the circus, because she learned he responded well to music earlier. "Oh, my, gosh—we put his TV music on old big band music. Benny Goodman came on playing *King Porter Stomp.* My grandfather used to play the piano and sing… When that song came on, he got up and started dancing, and he was just the happiest thing ever, so it was from that that I figured the old music calms him down. Oh, my, gosh—what a difference it made when you played music."[315]

Yvonne continued the music therapy, even after Richard's dancing days were behind him. "He would go through situations where he had pneumonia a couple of times. That was closer to the end of his life…so he'd have to stay at a rehab center, because he'd lose his legs a little bit, the muscles in his legs, and then he'd have to go through physical therapy before he could come home…He was in and out of rehab facilities. I had looked into the possibility of him staying somewhere for an extended time while I was going to take a vacation, but that never happened."[316] She smiled broadly again. "We ended up taking a vacation together. Out on the beach, there was a little cottage, because he used to always take us on vacations—take Grandpa on vacation. We didn't have to go far. We brought the dogs, we brought the cat, and there was a little cottage right on the beach, and the back porch—you see the ocean. He couldn't walk around, but he'd just sit out there and watch the dogs dig in the sand and look at the sunsets. It was beautiful."[317]

Her smile dimmed when her thoughts turned to her caregiver vigilance for keeping her grandfather safe at home. Nighttime was particularly unnerving for Yvonne. "He never opened the door, but he would never recognize that there was darkness in the house that means, 'I'm supposed to stay in bed.' He stopped realizing that…then he would go back to his bedroom after a little bit. I knew because I would hear him moving around. I didn't want to startle him, and I didn't want to take his independence away if he wanted to go out and sit in the living room for a couple of minutes because he was not sleeping. I was like, 'Okay—well, do that.' He got to the kitchen one night and he just started yelling that he was lost."[318]

"When he was losing more of his mobility, he started with a cane, then a walker, then a wheelchair. He didn't know to use his walker, so he was susceptible to falling. There were several occasions that he did fall, and that was pretty scary. Thank God he never broke anything. That never happened, but that was pretty scary."[319] A pause and a pained expression accompanied Yvonne's next comment. "He fell in the bathroom. The way he fell, his walker got caught. We couldn't get the door open to get to him…I logically knew it was not my fault, but to this day, I beat myself up over it. If I would have taken that bathroom door off, I could have gotten to him, and he wouldn't have been scared—He was scared."[320]

Yvonne recounted more of the caregiver routine and increased aide's presence she grew accustomed to for so long. "He was completely incontinent. I would change him in the middle of the night, but his bed, by the time he got up in the morning, would be wet, so that smell would be there. They had to make sure that they got all that cleaned up while he was going to the bathroom and then get him into the shower…They would have time to get the bed and all of that changed. Making sure that there was 'lazy food' in the house for him to eat was another concern."[321]

Before I could ask Yvonne to elaborate, she continued. "Lazy food. He did not like to chew, so if he could put it in his mouth and swallow it, he was good to go. However, he didn't like baby food. He didn't like anything that was not sweet…but then it got to a point where the doctor said that it's just the calories you have to worry about, so if he wants to eat ice cream six times a day, give him ice cream six times a day."[322]

When Yvonne finished explaining lazy food, she went back to describing daily caregiving life. "Even before I got out of bed, I had a camera that was facing his bed that when I opened my eyes when I woke up, the monitor was right there. I could tell whether or not he was in bed or he had fallen out of bed or whatever. That was always my first concern, 'Is Grandpa sleeping—in bed?' Then I would go in and just check on him. Then I would get into the shower. I'd have my coffee. The caregiver would come at 7:00. While I was getting dressed, they would go in and get him out of bed if he was going to wake up right then. Sometimes he did. Sometimes he didn't…I went from being able to be a private person to having people in my house all the time. I have OCD so I'd like things a certain way in my cabinets and stuff. I had to kind of let go of that and give up my privacy."[323]

Yvonne raised an eyebrow as she offered an example from when she was still trying to keep a full-time job and look after Richard. "Someone showed up early to do care. I used to have people come at 6:00 in the morning, and they would stay with him until 9. Then they would come back at 4 pm and stay with him until 6 when I got home. At 6 am, I would get up, and I would get my shower and go out and have my coffee. When someone just walks through your house at 6:15 and you're standing in the kitchen in your bathrobe—that's a challenge. One of the hardest things—I liked my utensils facing up. The caregiver just wouldn't do it…always facing down in the dishwasher. Just giving up those things that were mine, that was the biggest challenge. It's just your privacy."[324] She smiled, nodded her head and shared how she had dealt with it. "I could either spend my day upset about these stupid little things that I had no control over anymore, or I could say, 'Okay. This is just how it's going to be,' and that's what I did."[325]

She leaned back, took another long breath, and gazed past me as she walked herself back through her grandfather's progressive needs.

"I think my transitions, like from caregiving to medium to heavy, were so gradual. Like, it's like, if you were to dim the light, that's what I would compare it to. If you start dimming the light, and your eyes keep adjusting, you know? It was sort of like that because at first, it was just making the meals, cleaning, okay. Make sure the bills are paid, okay. Take him to the doctors' appointments, okay. Administer the medicine, handle all the shopping, okay. Handle all the finances, okay. Dress the grandpa, bathe the grandpa, but it was over the course of years that his deterioration was going. His Alzheimer's wasn't severe from Point A to Point B. It was in between, like slow losses of memory and what he could function and do for himself to what eventually he couldn't. I think maybe that gradualness to it allowed me to sort of adjust with what I was doing as a caregiver. Does that make sense? In the beginning...I didn't understand everything about Alzheimer's. I didn't really know anything about it. I would try to reason with him and stuff, but as I started getting more information, little bit more educated or talking to other people that went through it, I was like, 'Oh, okay. This is what to expect. He's not going to understand certain things and that's okay, just keep the atmosphere peaceful and calm, and stay loving and kind and that will keep him peaceful.'"[326]

She looked back at the makeshift memorial on the table, her eyes drawn to those of her grandfather in one of the photos. "He didn't always know who I was. Even then, when he looked at me, he knew that he loved me, but he didn't quite know why. When he stopped calling me by my name." Yvonne looked up to tell me why Richard's not remembering her name was so hard on her. "He named me. My name was supposed to be Constance. He told my mother that I was 'too pretty of a baby to name her Constance,' so my mother told my grandfather, 'You name her.' He named me Yvonne, so he loved my name. Up until a dozen years ago, he was the only person that called me Yvonne. Everybody always called me Eve, and I hate Eve. I like Yvonne. He stopped using my name. That's when I really started seeing him start to go downhill even more."[327] Tears pooled in Yvonne's eyes as she lightly pressed her fingertips to the glass over Richard's printed image. "When I'd be there, and he just looked through me and didn't know who I was—I just wanted him to, please, just say, 'I love you.'"[328]

Final Horizon

Fred glanced down at Princess, still sleeping by his feet, then sighed and told me having Mary in a facility is what's best for both him and his wife. "We see our friends who just beat themselves to death trying to care at home for the loved one—thinking that they're doing best. Many, many times they find out that they've tried to do more than they should have done and it really wasn't good enough… They're doing it out of love and yet, their love is not the best thing for their loved one anymore."[329]

He still seemed lonely, but described his mindset on being the well person at home for a spouse in a memory care unit. "I believe that, if they are at a facility, you yourself have to just not curl up in a chair and feel sorry for yourself and think, 'Well, maybe if I had done this or done that. Oh, I'll watch TV or something.' You still have to be motivated enough to get out. Whether it's church, a club, golf, the gym….I go to SilverSneakers® [330]…three times a week. And where I live, there's a little club right around the corner…I don't like to go down and just sit at the bar, but I go down and I like to hear the music—and the support group meeting and stuff like that."[331] He smiled when he said, "I told somebody at the gym that I was an 'octogenarian' now and they told me they were 'Presbyterian!'…I try to keep my sense of humor. Humor and music. I like to listen to music late in the afternoon, have a martini then have my dinner."[332]

Fred finished his thought as he looked back down at his cat. "So I try to stay involved with some of these things, but then one person maintaining a house, and even though it's a little cat, it still takes time. You have double the work when it's just you and what to do."[333]

I found my own gaze had followed Fred's down toward Princess, so I asked him how Mary interacted with their cat when she was still at home. "She loved the cat and, when she was still in rehab, I took Princess over a couple of times—but then it scared Princess because she wanted to hold her and she held her pretty tight…Since that, I have not tried to take her…and she hasn't brought it up. I don't want to remind her and, 'Oh, where is she?'"[334] Fred's visits now consisted of his going to the facility by himself and seeing her there—without leaving the complex together. "I can't take her out anymore, because I have nobody to make sure I can handle her."[335]

He used to feel bad leaving her behind, because when he'd try to leave, he said she'd say, "'I want to go home. I want to leave this place.' I explained to her that she's there because she's 'had to take the medicine to help her brain out.' She said, 'We can do that at home.' She's got an answer."[336] "You have to be very careful of what you say, and I found out in leaving. It used to be, 'Oh, I have to go now. I have to go out and stop at the store.' 'Oh, I'll go with you and I'll stay in the car.' And if I'd just say, 'I have to go.' 'Well I'll go with you.'… then you have to try to work your way out of that. So, what I did, if she said, 'Where are you going?' I'd say, 'At the office, I need some papers I have to sign.' 'Okay,' that's understood. A 'medical fib' now and then. You have to work with it. Whatever keeps them calm."[337]

Fred gave another medical fib example to show he wasn't the only one at the facility to use them. "There's a lady there that, every time I go down about 1:00 or so, she comes to the door that's the lock-down section, and she's rolled up some sweaters and stuff in a ball, and she stands there with them and the aide. She'll say she's waiting for her brother or husband or something that's gonna pick her up—and she stands there and waits. Then they'll come over and say, 'They called—there's a part missing in his car and they have to get the part from the factory—so he's not going to be able to make it today.' She'll say, 'Okay.' So she goes back to her room. And they do this almost every day. The same thing. A medical fib. It satisfies her and rather than saying, 'Oh, well he's not coming.' And, 'Oh, well the part hasn't come in yet.' The part hasn't come in now in over a year, but it's a nice way to handle it."[338]

Fred appeared partially comforted having seen the facility's staff calmly attend to Mary and her fellow memory impaired patients. "If a resident gets upset for one reason or another, they'll come over and they'll hold their hands and embrace them and talk to them. Just whispering to them pretty much and sort of trying to just distract them is what it amounts to. They don't hesitate, they just don't hesitate to do that kind of thing. I've seen them do it with Mary and I've seen them do it with so many of the others."[339]

Fred said the support group opinions differ on visiting a spouse in a memory care unit. "There's two philosophies that I hear…these facilities, some of them want you to not visit your spouse for like two weeks—and basically what they're doing is trying to get that person to forget who the spouse was, so they're taking commands and information from them—and I've heard some bad stories from people that come here that have gone through that. Then the other is, if you keep coming, they're dependent upon you."[340]

He said Mary's not always very receptive when he stops in to see her. "I sometimes aggravate her when I visit her. Just walking in. She would, 'What are you doing here?' 'Well, I came to visit you.' 'Well, you were here yesterday.' Well, actually I wasn't. 'Well, I can visit you twice, can't I?' She'd try to tell you something and then couldn't finish the sentence. And whatever she was trying to tell you wasn't coherent anyway…and it would really upset her that she couldn't finish the sentence. So, I learned not to ask her anything. You know, 'What are you doing?' or 'Do you remember so and so?' At that point, they don't remember and it causes them to really get upset to try to."[341] "She is pretty alert in the morning, but then as the day progresses, she regresses and sometimes gets a little bit of rough behavior, I would say, or tries to. You have to watch what you say to her or she'll really jump all over you."[342]

Fred said he visits less frequently than when Mary first went in two years ago. "I just go down and make sure…I find it very important to make sure everybody knows you're there and learn the names and talk to them. I think it's very good to know the people…taking care of her…in the facility…If there's any kind of an incident, they do call me right away. Then of course, I go down."

Once again Fred seemed to be scanning my face for an expression for approval, or not, of his visitation frequency. Seeing neither, he continued, "I could go down every day and sit there for ten minutes, but there's really nobody to talk to and then she gets a little aggravated too, so I just go down and talk to her a little bit."[343] In a melancholy tone, Fred admitted, "She doesn't respond to too much. I give her a hug or something and she kind of… If you want just a brief acknowledgement any way which is good, but it's hard to say anything because it's hard for it to register as to what I'm saying. I try to keep my sentences as short as possible. You don't want long drawn out…because after a few words, they know a little bit about what you're saying. If it's a big long sentence, they just tune you out. They can't follow it."[344]

While Mary can't carry on conversations anymore, Fred noted the other visitors who still try to look in on her. "People from our church, about four or five different women, come up and see my wife and visit her. The pastor comes up there. He was just up there this past Thursday. I think that's helping her. As far as a social life, that's all the social life she gets… Tomorrow I'm going to take her to the beauty shop. Hopefully, I can take her to the beauty shop. Her hair's getting sort of long, so I want to get it cut short and make it easier to take care of her here. I hope that works. The last time we went, it worked out just fine."[345]

He hesitated for a moment, then said, "They had to Baker Act her. She got violent and was throwing glasses at people, was trying to claw them with her fingernails and stuff…something really set her off. So, she was probably there for close to a week and then she went back to the facility. They adjusted her medicine, and that seemed to have calmed her down then quite a bit. But every now and then, she doesn't do that now, but once in a while, she gets feisty. And if she says, 'No!' and when she raises her eyes, she's got brown eyes, when she raises those eyes, you better back off! And they've all learned that."[346]

Fred smiled when he gave an example of Mary's feistiness. "They told me when she was in the dining room that they had a new girl that was just there temporarily…She kept trying to give Mary this glass of water or something and…she said, 'No, I don't want it.' She said, 'Take this glass of water!' And the other aides were having problems with this new girl too. I don't know if she was new, but she was new to that section. And she (Mary) said, 'Okay.' She took the glass of water and she threw it in her face—and the aides told me they wanted to applaud. I'd love to have done that myself. Yeah, that was great."[347]

As Fred's somewhat prideful expression waned, he offered his final thought on Mary's facility. "I think maybe they're giving her too much medicine, because…she wasn't that way when she went in there. Either the brain is vastly deteriorating, or it's the medicine. It's got to be one or the other…They've got their own doctor over there, some psychiatrist prescribed a bunch of stuff for my wife."[348]

I asked Fred if he had put a safety net[349] into place, in case something happened to him while Mary was still alive. His response came almost immediately. "I'm not too concerned about that, because I have everything—a will prepared. My daughter is very—I've educated her to what my desires are. I have paperwork in place to do— for her to be able to do this. I have an emergency list for my neighbors if something happens to me. They have a copy of what to do, who to call, and what to do for my wife, in the short term."[350] "If I died, she would come down here and take her out of the home, and take her up there and try to find something up there."[351]

Fred told me Alzheimer's had been in the family before Mary. I asked if that was also a subject discussed with their daughter. "I have talked to our daughter about the possibility of testing. Genetic testing I guess it would be. I think she's adverse to that because if she does test positive, or whatever the term is, I think they would be extremely disappointed and probably very scared about what the future might hold, even though it might not come to fruition. I can respect that. I don't know that I would do anything different now if that choice were offered to me."[352] Fred slowed his speech in a slightly lowered tone. "I knew that her mother had it and everything, and I never…I guess I put it in the back of my mind, 'My wife isn't going to get that.' Now, I look at… 'My girl might get it. My girl's sons might get it.' I don't understand why this happens. That's the thing. I don't understand why it happens. What do we do wrong in order to get our brain to shrink? I can see hardening of the arteries. I can see that, because of things you eat and everything can cause something like that. The dementia, I don't understand that. I never will."[353]

As we neared the end of our interview, I asked Fred what caregiver fears he had for his cognitively impaired wife, Mary. "I don't want her to do something to get hurt...as most people don't die from dementia, they're gonna die from something else—and that can come very quickly if they get something or they fall—that can cause complications."[354] "They had me sign a paper saying, 'If she gets to that point, do you want us to use a feeding tube in the side?' And I talked to one of the management people from an insurance group that they have. She said, 'I can't tell you what to do.' But she said, 'Usually, that's not a good idea because they get infections and it's just a poor way to...and she wouldn't want that anyway.' So, we rejected that idea. If she gets to that point, why keep postponing it and postponing it and postponing it and postponing it? When there's no life there—there's just nothing there."[355]

Upon hearing his own words, Fred sounded desperate for approval. "We have been married 56 years, we've had a good relationship and I know I don't deserve it, but a lot of people here say, 'You really do a good job with her.' I know I'm not doing a great job, but I'm doing what I can."[356] Fred's eyes filled with tears as he struggled to finish, "Having...I'm sorry...Seeing her in the home—can't do nothing about it...I'm sorry."[357] I told Fred it was okay, that he didn't have to keep going, but he shook his head and finally squeaked out, "Send her to heaven... That's her thought, 'I want to go to heaven.'"[358]

* * *

"It's very traumatizing, I mean—the bedroom door would be shut and I would think, 'I need to be quiet, George's in there.' And then I had to say, 'No, he's not.' And it's a big adjustment. If I didn't have a pet—I would be in mental anguish—but I have to take care of her and I still have to be a little caregiver. So...it's good that I have her."[359] Momentarily, Janice's grief overtook her. I handed her another tissue and asked if she wanted us to pause the interview. "No. I'm pretty strong. I'm pretty strong,"[360] she said, through her tears. "I knew I'd be in it for the long haul. I knew I'd have to get help. I knew that. I knew that you can't do this type of thing all, totally, on your own. I also journaled throughout the whole seven years, and in the margins, I would either put a smiley face, a flat face, or sad, or tears, and it helped me going back, after he passed, to see how strong I was, and how much I did, because you don't think you can do this kind of stuff. You really don't."[361]

She had finished wiping her eyes. "You have years of marriage, and it's a give and take, and good and bad, and then all of a sudden, for me to become the controller, or the caregiver—I guess I was kind of surprised that he didn't balk at it more. Once he accepted it, he accepted it very well, except when he'd get upset, frustrated, but—his intention was not to harm anybody. It was the frustration. It was just confusion, and I did let him know, 'I'm here for you. I will be here. You've been a good husband. Right now, you're not feeling well.'… I'm not sure what he understood, but I would hold his hand a lot."[362] "If he didn't know who I was, he knew I was the one that would take care of him. He knew that."[363]

"He changed,"[364] Janice said contemplatively. "You know, here he was the…first 12 years of our marriage…extremely, extremely good looking, full of himself, fun loving, very self-centered, narrow minded, but generous. Generous with the things that he wanted to be generous with, like, 'Come on, let's go out to eat.' 'Oh here, I'm going to get a new car. I'll give you my old one.' Now meantime, he had…a company car…whenever he needed to go someplace. You know, all this. It was always a little, 'Yeah, that's a great car you have, but buy me something new.' I always—You remember when the commercials came out about the Mercedes with the red bows on them for Christmas? I always thought one day he would do that for me, and he never did. Somewhere during his disease—he became very unfiltered. He lost all this macho…and he became—not child-like, he never became child-like—but he became so gentle and kind. It was like a gift."[365]

Her thoughts turned back to their dog. "I don't rely on people, but I was an only child. So, I have always been, I'll say, content to be alone. I mean, I don't mind. I mean, it's why I got the dog. I got her about a year and a half before George passed, because I knew. We didn't have a dog for years because we were working, and it's really not fair to have—So, I knew. I mean, you could see the handwriting on the wall that I was going to be alone. So, I got the dog, and she's been a lifesaver."[366]

Reminding herself that she wasn't alone seemed to buoy her resolve to finish telling me about her experience with George. "I put him in an assisted living…and I think, I think he gave up. I really do. I think in his non-mind, it was a different place, it was a different routine. He ate some, but not too much, and all he wanted to do was sit, and I was upset. He ended up getting quite a big bed sore, and with hospice and the assisted living, that shouldn't of happened, but they asked me what I wanted to do, and I said, 'Just keep him comfortable,' because I knew he wasn't coming back."

"I mean, physically, we could've healed the sore, but it was bad. It was really bad. I was surprised, but they told me, hospice told me, that when the body starts to break down, it can break down pretty fast, because he was not up and walking. But we were putting him in chairs and moving him around, and he was, to my mind, okay a few days before I noticed the bad bed sore, but when it starts to break down, it does."[367]

I watched Janice as she recalled and shared what had happened only a few weeks before our interview. She pressed on, without pauses, to allow herself to get through it. "Well, he had contracted pneumonia…They sent him to the hospital…I was going to go that night to see him…I talked to the guy, and he said, 'Don't bother.' He said, 'He's fine. We're doing fine. You can come tomorrow. You know he'll probably be in the room.' On my way out there, I thought, 'Well, I'll check with the home to see what I have to do, if anything.' I hadn't gone through this before. 'Don't worry. He's back.' I said, 'What?' Well, they said he has pneumonia and he's on antibiotics. They said he's going to be fine. I said, 'But I was told'—She said, 'Well, they sent him back.'"[368]

With her head shaking, Janice continued. "All that week he had been very tired and coughing. I had mentioned it to the nurse. She said, 'Well, we'll check into it'…Nothing was done…that was Friday. Saturday I went out and he wasn't feeling too good. I went to church

Sunday—of course, I was usually at my church. I turned my phone off. I didn't get home until one or so. On the phone was a message that they had taken George to the hospital.… That was late in the afternoon…I was going out, and I called the ALF to let them know that he was going to be there for two or three days. 'He's back.' I said, 'What?'"[369]

Janice said George still didn't show any signs of improvement. "He wouldn't eat. He still had this, whatever it was, at that time. They said pneumonia. They said it was gone a week before, but it was back again. It was really bad, so they sent him to the hospital…Well come to find out, what he had was what they call aspirational pneumonia. The brain evidently doesn't do it. Everything was shutting down… The next day, Dr. Oscher was his doctor. I was on my way out. He said, 'Don't come. We're going to be putting him in ICU. He'll be there until we can decide what's going on. You can come anytime tomorrow you want, anytime. Just let us get him settled tonight.' I went that night, or that next day and talked to Dr. Oscher. He said he had a kidney infection, or his urine was the color of cocoa. He had things in his nose, in his throat, in his backside, everywhere… He talked to me about signing a DNR, which we have a DNR or had one. In order for them to not resuscitate, I had to sign another paper with this doctor."[370]

Janice sat bedside as the hospital staff tended to George. "I can't say enough about the ICU. They were wonderful to me as well as him."[371] She added, "He grabbed my hand. In a comatose state, he grabbed my hand really, really hard. I was so scared, I pulled my hand away. It wasn't until maybe a week later, I said, 'Oh, God, maybe he just wanted to hang on and say good-bye,' and I was afraid. I was afraid, and so I pulled away. You know, I don't beat myself up for these sort of things that you do out of instinct. I know, in my heart, I did my best. I don't have any guilt."[372]

"I remember when he died. I just felt such a tremendous sense of relief—because it isn't just physically, it was responsibly. I made every single decision here about the house, about our life, about finances, about my health, his health, everything. I dealt with… everything. I got to the point where, oh my God, I was exhausted with everything and when he died, I knew that was done."[373] "Seven years is a long time to get used to the idea that you're saying goodbye. For seven years you're saying goodbye. You're saying goodbye to every little thing about that person is gone."[374]

She finally paused for an extended moment—tears welling again. "Tell you the truth, that's the hardest thing I've ever done in my life and it will be the hardest thing I ever do, is taking care of him—because you see somebody that you love degenerate right before your eyes. They're gone. And he was such an intelligent man. Our relationship started based on just talking for hours about everything and so, to lose that partner, that was hard…I miss having him there to talk to…his companionship. I love him and I just miss him. That was hard to see that go. I wish it had gone in a better way. I'd rather say goodbye to somebody that died of something other than Alzheimer's where you're not really saying—you said goodbye so many times, it's in the past."[375]

"I guess I'd do it again. I'd do the same thing. I don't know if I would even contemplate…a home. I think I'd probably…get somebody to come in 24 hours or whatever they had to do…then, stay home…I did not like people coming into my home. I didn't enjoy that one bit, but you do what you got to do." Janice dabbed at her eyes again, focused intensely on mine and said, "I did get to be with him when he drew his last breath and for some reason, that was important to me. I told him I'd be there 'til the end and I was."[376]

* * *

Alice said in the four months Audrey was in the lockdown ward, she did her best to stave off her mother's family memories from disappearing completely. "I put photos and other information of all of her family members all over…so that she could turn and see them throughout the decline. Towards the end, she mostly just stayed in bed and slept…My husband and I made it a point not to correct her if she got anything wrong, not to worry if she did anything unusual that wasn't dangerous, and to listen attentively and actively, no matter how many times she repeated anything…There were stories that we must have heard innumerable times, but we had promised our-selves that we would deal with this and we did. It was good. So many people often are trying to correct the thoughts or patterns of their relative who is going through this, not realizing that it's not going to make a difference one way or another. I did my best to agree with Mother when some of these memory gaps came up and just allow that to move forward."[377]

Audrey's decline soon involved far more than her fading memory. "The day my mother fell down, she broke her hip, she shattered her hip actually, and her knee just popped out…She survived…and then she had a total cognitive impairment. She would not know what she was talking about. She would not know if she was sleeping. She could not pee, poop…I mean, she was kind of lost. At that time, she was just a person living but not living."[378]

"I was at the facility…and I asked…'What is the procedure when eventually the person passes away?' She says, 'Well, we call you and you have the decision to make if you want to come down once the person has passed away and stay with the body…or if you don't want to come and we just wait for the funeral home.' I said, 'Well, what do most people do?' She said, 'Well, truthfully most people come, but most of the people that come feel guilty that they haven't been there, so now they feel they need to come…There were some that never visited and then there were some that always visited.' She said, 'The ones that never visited are the first to show up when you call them when the person has died.'"[379]

"She just basically died just like many people with this disease. They stop taking nourishment and all and just pass away."[380] Alice was wringing her hands as her eyes were fixed on the table before her. "They just said, 'Look, we can't do anything, we're going to make her comfortable.' So hospice took over."[381] "We were—when she took her last breath—we were all in the room with her. We never made the decision what would we do, and my children are like, 'I don't know if I want my last memory to come and see her lying there having passed away.' It never came to that because we were there the whole day when she did pass away."[382]

Alice stayed silent for a long moment, then looked up to make sure I was still listening intently before she returned to speaking. "The other thing with Alzheimer's is there's a grieving process. With other diseases, you grieve mostly when the person has died. If the loved one has a heart attack and heart disease or diabetes, but their mind is still sharp, the grieving process usually begins later or even after death. But with Alzheimer's, first you lose this intellectual person that you can have a conversation with."[383]

She said despite having started the grieving process early, she was too weary to speak at Audrey's memorial service. While she didn't share what the pastor or her siblings said at the church, she smiled— though still teary-eyed—to tell me about Bill speaking at her mother's post-service reception. "After her death, my husband stood and then he talked about me, how I helped her and how she would just listen to me because I was the one. That gave me strength, that made me happy. It made me satisfied…that people were aware because not everybody was aware. At that time, it just made me happy that I was there for her to help her through and that it was recognized."[384]

Her comfort for having dutifully completed her tasks for Audrey was short-lived. "After my mother passed…my brother was kind of assuming the role of the executor of the estate, but years before that, he had come here. They had met with an attorney. They came back. The attorney said, 'We need all this stuff.' So I got all the stuff. All of it. Every single life insurance policy, every single stock, every single everything, and I left my brother a three-page note that says, 'This is what you need to do.' He said, 'Yeah, yeah, yeah, I'll do it.' He didn't do it. So none of the beneficiary stuff got changed. My brother had assumed certain things would happen. Well, they didn't happen. So things didn't get changed."[385]

Alice spoke in an exasperated tone as to the consequences for her brother's failure to do his part previously. "My dad and my mom had wills drawn up by my father's friend who also was a very clever real estate attorney and had no clue how to do an appropriate will, apparently. My dad left everything to my mom. My mom left everything to my dad. There wasn't any mention of us even though we were there because it was in the 1980's. We got to the estate attorney, and he said, 'These are pretty much worthless.' Although it was clever, he got it all done on one page. They were totally worthless. We had to prove we were the only offspring of my parents."[386]

"Everybody decided, my brother, my sisters…that I take over as the administrator of the estate. I was able to get probably 90% of it done within that first year, and then there were some odds and ends that were such a pain."[387] I sensed that Alice seemed mad at both the process and being the sibling that took on the final chore by herself. "Probate's a pain. I know why probate has to exist. It's just ridiculous how long it takes. I mean, it took me two years to settle my mom's estate."[388]

"Even the house, when we moved her into assisted living, it took us almost a year of squeezing it in around work getting her house cleaned out, because my mom was a saver. It was organized and…she had 57 boxes of Christmas decorations! She had decorations for every holiday and this was an entire lifetime of stuff of hers that we had to deal with that they didn't seem to understand that was a huge undertaking for us."[389] Alice said they still had most of Audrey's things when she died. "We had a 10' x 24' storage facility rented because we didn't have room for all of her keepsakes at our house and…to her…those things were her life…Her stuff meant the world to her."[390] Alice and Bill had protected Audrey's keepsakes throughout her years in assisted living and the memory care unit so she could still enjoy them. "We had an air-conditioned storage facility and during the holidays, we'd sneak over there and grab a couple of her totes to use some of her decorations."[391]

Once she took over as her mother's executrix, Alice expected her siblings would appreciate that she had preserved Audrey's keepsakes so they could each choose their own mementos. A scowl emerged on Alice's face as she described what, to her, had been their final insult to Audrey. "'Throw it all out!' I think, that in their mind, it was as easy as, 'Take everything of Mom's and get rid of it'…So the thought that they just said, 'Have somebody come and pick it all up and take it all away'—I think that was the most upsetting to me."[392]

* * *

Picking up the large white photo frame, Yvonne cleared her throat to tell me how Richard's Alzheimer's journey ended. "He was never in a long-term facility as far as staying there. He stayed at home and really his wish was to pass at home…his body was just shutting down."[393] "He had a major stroke and…was sent to the hospital. Yeah, so we went in and he literally couldn't talk, couldn't swallow."[394] "And he clearly stated in his living will, once he was in a condition where his organs were shutting down, he wasn't able to eat, he didn't want his life sustained indefinitely without the recovery to happen….The doctors were very, very kind…I read his whole living will and I said, 'He's not here to speak for himself.' I was his advocate at that point, so I said, 'I'm going to read this. This is his voice,' and read through the whole thing."[395] "He had signed his living will. He did not want to be resuscitated, but his thing that he always said to me—because my grandmother had died actually in the hospital and he was there and it was horrible—and he always said to me, 'Honey, don't ever let me die in a hospital or a nursing home. I want to go home. Will you take me home?'"[396]

I watched Yvonne move Richard's framed portrait to her lap, which she gently cradled while speaking. "So, when he had the stroke and they're telling me there's nothing that they could do…I looked at my boyfriend and my minister lady friend and I said, 'We need to take him home.' They said, 'Yvonne, that's 24-hour care!' I said, 'Okay.' 'You can't do this by yourself.' I said, 'Nope, I can't. But, I'll tell you what—if we take him home, I think we'll have friends that will come. I think I'll get help, and if I don't get help, I'll do it.' They just looked at me… So…I looked at the doctor, I said, 'That's what we need to do,' and he's like, 'Well, you can send hospice to the house.' When they wheeled him in, in his foyer area, he had his mounted bass that he had caught. They were masterpieces. He was a good fisherman. So, as they wheeled him in, he literally had tears running down the side of his face…That, right there, told me that he knew he was home. So, he had tears running down his face, and I think he recognized every single person that was there, just by his eyes…We all agreed that we would be there the whole entire time. Hospice comes in, sets everything up, and we…didn't want anybody to overdose him on anything, so we made out a med list basically of when we're doing the morphine, where everybody checked it off and did everything, because we were taking turns. Hospice was just amazed."[397]

Yvonne stopped and asked me if I had been in Florida when a hurricane had crossed the state. I nodded, vividly remembering the year hurricanes Charley, Frances, Jeanne, and Ivan all hit Florida within just 48 days. Her speech picked up speed as Yvonne continued. "Then, a hurricane was coming…So, they said, 'We can't stay here, and you have the option of moving him to the hospice house, or if you guys decide to stay home, then hospice care cannot be here.' So, I said, 'He wanted to be home. Just a Category 1 hurricane,[398] I think we're going to be fine.' My minister and everybody agreed that that should be fine, Category 1, not a big deal, in most cases not a big deal. Anyways, the nurse said to me, she goes, 'I don't understand why he's hanging on. Typically, somebody with the level of stroke that he's had would've already been gone.' She's like, 'The only thing I can think of there's got to be some type of date, anniversary date, coming up of somebody in the family that's close to him,' and I was like, 'Oh, my birthday's the 1st, but that's still a ways.' She's like, 'Yeah, he's not going to last until the 1st.' She goes, 'But,' she says, 'I'm just going to go ahead and tell you.' She says, 'A lot of times people die on special events for a reason, and that's because that person is special to them. He's probably not going to die on your birthday, but there's a big chance he could be buried on your birthday. Are you okay with that?' I was like, 'Oh, my God.' She's like, 'Just remember, if it happens, it's because you meant a lot to him.' It's like, 'Oh, my God.' I, of course, didn't think anything of it."[399]

"The hurricane comes through…when you're in the moment of a caregiver and somebody's dying!"[400] Yvonne's eyes widened with an alarmed look as her voice maintained the swift pace. "I don't understand—his oxygen—he ran out of oxygen! My grandfather ran out— he was running out of oxygen! We had no power. Power was gone. My boyfriend gets in the pickup truck, goes to the neighbor down the street…in the middle of the hurricane, to go get a generator so we could have oxygen for my grandfather. I sit back, going, 'Oh, my, gosh—he risked his life!' Because at this point, the storm was pretty massive and he did, we got the generator, and we were able to get there and get everything going so he had his oxygen. That's pretty much the only thing we did, could barely run that and the lamp in there with him. Then, once he passed and we had the windows open, there was like this big swoop of wind, and it was actually the eye of the hurricane passing over. This wind just goes right through. I mean, literally you could feel it as he passed. It was almost like, I felt like the angels had come and took him."[401]

Pausing for a moment to take a deeper look at her grandfather's face in the photo, Yvonne's speech cadence returned to a calming tone. "He passed. The hurricane came. He had his funeral arrangements to be made at Eternal Memorial Gardens. Hurricane came, blew the roof off of Eternal Memorial Gardens. My minister was trying to get funeral arrangements made up, and they're saying they can't accommodate, when that's where my grandfather wanted it. My minister says, 'They can't schedule anything.' I said, 'That's insane!' I said, 'I don't care if we have to stand by the grave side! I don't care what they do!' She goes, 'You know what? You're absolutely right, Honey.' My minister…called them up and says, 'Everything's paid for at your facility. We are not going anywhere else to have this funeral. I want you to get with your head director, whoever it may be, and tell them this funeral service needs to be scheduled there at Eternal Memorial Gardens, and I want you to call me back within the next hour and give me the date and time you are going to accommodate us. I don't care if you have to pitch a tent or what you have to do to accommodate my grandfather. I want it done.' The guy says, 'What a great idea. We can get a tent. Let me see what we can do about that.' He calls me back and says, 'October 1st at 10:00 in the morning, we will accommodate your family.' That was my birthday, my 33rd birthday. I felt almost kind of upset it was my birthday, but then I also, because of what the hospice nurse had shared with me, kind of had a little bit of joy knowing, because I did take care of him. So, in the end, I think that was his way of saying thank you."[402]

Yvonne's eyes glistened, yet she was smiling. Still holding Richard's portrait, she seemed glad she had been able to share their story aloud. She slowly scanned each of the photos on the table, then offered a final reflection on her caregiving experience. "I think there was a very decisive moment in time when I did look at the situation and say, 'I'm right where I want to be, right where I need to be, right where I'm supposed to be. I'm going to see this thing out.' I had a deep desire to honor the one who took responsibility for me when my parents didn't. Yeah, so it was a privilege really."[403]

Researcher's Note

As each of the interview participants finished sharing their own family caregiving experience, I thanked them for their openness. They unanimously thanked me back—for listening and wanting to draw more attention to the subject. I welcomed them to give advice to future caregivers, family members, friends, neighbors, doctors, employers, politicians, or whoever they wished had better understood their perspective—believing their insight might best inform on the phenomenon. When they were done—I turned off the audio recorder for a post-interview discussion.

I thanked them again, saying I hoped they had found the interview cathartic, and reminded them of the local support group contacts—if they desired further discussion for any unresolved items. Earlier, in the pre-interview consent form review, I had already told them their personal stories and advice would be blended into a research-informed book, written in a nonacademic voice for a public audience.

In the post-interview debriefing, I no longer had to guard against influencing their responses. Having held strongly to all the research protocols needed to ensure the data collected would accurately reflect their experiences, I could now tell them the book's motivation stemmed from my decades of personal and professional connections to Alzheimer's and dementia—and my grave concern for the looming wave of cognitively impaired baby boomers. They thanked me for sharing, more fully realizing the importance of their participation ahead of the crisis they would help me illuminate.

Rock 'n' Roll to Rocking Chairs

Storm Warning

Researcher's Note

For young children living in Florida, car rides to Orlando are usually a joyous occasion—for that is where Mickey Mouse lives and so many other fantastic family adventures take place. But in the 1960s, there were no theme parks for us to enjoy—just mile after mile and hours of bumpy interstate highway that we traveled upon to reach my grandparents.

As a child, I did not understand seeing my father's pale face and exhausted posture when he would usher me and my sister back into the car to drive home. I was oblivious to the effort my mother was making to keep us quiet whenever he went into his mother's room at her nursing home. No, my memories of my grandmother were wonderful—playing by her side in the living room or sneaking a snack in the kitchen. I have no recall of her fading away from the family—but my parents did. My Mamaw's dementia type may not have been officially identified then— but that did not matter.

That was the first time a dementia ailment touched my life—and I did not even know to be concerned. I did not know how my grandmother's illness affected her physically. I did not know the emotional toil it brought for those around her—my parents, my sister, my aunts, my uncles, and my cousins. I knew nothing of the medical decisions, financial difficulties, legal challenges, family dynamic stresses, or the extended impact it had on everyone's work.

No one ever spoke of my grandmother's ailment, as such was simply not done. I was a child, so I was spared from reality—but I grew up.

* * *

For many generations, families have silently dealt with Alzheimer's, dementia, or other cognitive impairment. As my generation, the baby boomers, grow older, there will be far more occurrences. There are over 5.5 million Americans currently living with Alzheimer's, with that total expected to climb to an estimated 13.8 to 16 million afflicted individuals by 2050.[404]

In a country of over 300 million people, some may be inclined to simply do the math and say, "The odds are I won't get it," then turn their attention to more pleasant things. However, as the caregiver stories in "Love Thy Stranger" have just demonstrated, those *afflicted* by Alzheimer's or dementia are not the only ones *affected* by it.

In fact, the upward trend in the incidence of Alzheimer's and dementia cases in the United States should elevate the number of unpaid family caregivers to an estimated 40 to 46 million.[405] Do the math again, and most people will realize that in some fashion, they will likely be affected by the wave of cognitively impaired baby boomers. Such a sizable percentage of the population being directly affected means that nearly everyone will become personally aware of someone acting in a caregiver role. Yet the math offers no advance knowledge to them of who that personally-known caregiver will be. Perhaps it will be their coworker, their neighbor, their friend, a family member—or themselves.

Individuals and families must become keenly aware of how their personal resources and support systems may change before they find themselves either afflicted or affected by Alzheimer's or dementia. Awareness and discussion over the responsibilities and abilities for families or governments to handle the costs of caring for the cognitively impaired baby boomers are also highly warranted.

Medicare and Medicaid may require reforms to stay solvent as the elder population swells. Those changes will surely impact federal and state governments, but also a wide spectrum within the health care industry—from doctors, nurses, and other care providers, to insurers, pharmaceuticals, and care products. All these segments would be wise to candidly assess their options to plan and make adjustments in advance of this wave, because by 2050, every 33 seconds, someone in the United States will develop Alzheimer's.[406]

Families, industry, and government also need to be aware that this wave will carry a total of over $10 trillion of wealth being controlled by individuals "without legal capacity" by 2050.[407] Protecting the elderly against the possibility of an exponential increase in financial exploitation will require advanced planning and safeguards.

Fortunately, it is by advanced analysis, discussion, and action that large challenges may be lessened or even circumvented. If the folk wisdom, "A stitch in time saves nine," is too subtle a reminder for some—let them recall the business axiom, "Those who fail to plan, plan to fail." Simple as these statements may be, both are intended as empowering messages. Individuals, government, and industry can each choose to better assess their potential future needs to consider how best to get ready for the changes ahead.

There are numerous socioeconomic and government level areas deserving study ahead of the aging of the baby boomers. This research-informed book's "unit of analysis"[408] is at the individual family level. At the center of the coming crisis will be the millions of cognitively impaired individuals and their family caregivers.

> *"I didn't realize this until I picked up the death report when she was cremated. I picked up her remains and the death report. I really felt bad that they didn't say she died of Alzheimer's or Parkinson's because that's how funding is determined. Federal funding, if nobody dies from it, you don't get—No money goes into it."*[409]

* * *

> *"The silence that goes along with recognition of this disease needs to be—the disease needs to be more out front. More okay for people to have.*
>
> *If somebody comes in and says, 'I have cancer,' and you go, 'Oh, I'm so sorry. What part of your body do you have cancer in? How bad is it?'*
>
> *I would like for somebody to say—be able to say, 'Well, I have dementia. Dementia comes in a lot of different forms. Let me tell you about my demen-tia…one of these days I'm not gonna be as good as I am now…So, I want you to know and I want you*

*to be my friend. I want you to stay with me until I
can't be.*"[410]

As in the research participants' quotes above, the caregivers in this study wanted their messages to be heard—to help, to heal, and to prepare those who will be at the epicenter of the millions upon millions of cognitively impaired baby boomers and their family caregivers. "Love Thy Stranger" shared candid caregiver experiences in their own words to help readers better contemplate their own future connection to the looming wave of cognitive impairment identified in "Rock 'n' Roll to Rocking Chairs." A research method described in "Behind the Curtain" explains how "Fred," "Janice," "Alice," and "Yvonne" became the four names and representative faces chosen to present the words voiced by the study's 24 actual caregivers in the case stories. Study participants' firsthand insights and "Researcher's Notes" continue informing throughout each of these chapters, with "Research Reflections" providing lesson reminders, "Caregivers' Advice," and thoughts on their "Own Cognitive Impairment."

This book applauds the vital and valiant scientific efforts being made to combat this disease, but it will focus upon the expanding "stakeholder impact"[411]—those who may be affected beyond the afflicted themselves. In my childhood example, my grandmother's relatives, their children, their employers, etc. are considered to have been "stakeholders" to her ailment. Some were direct, others more indirect, but all were affected in some manner. The research study's caregiver participants' own words have provided some semblance of their direct stakeholder impact from their family member's cognitive impairment. Like ripples on a pond, those impacts extend outward—usually diminishing the further they are away from the center. Yet similar to the physical properties of wave effects—the emotional, financial, and lasting family or work implications may impact the layers of direct and indirect caregiving stakeholders differently. Imagine a sturdy boat's ease in rolling over a swell, while some shorelines can suffer erosion—simply by being gnawed away from a constant lapping of minor waves.

As these baby boomers age, Alzheimer's and dementia will not remain an ailment in the shadows—far away from those who were previously unaffected. The study's caregivers agreed that if empathy for those impacted helped create an awareness of the problem, then awareness of the problem itself could potentially provoke action. Storm preparation is best done before the skies have darkened.

Researcher's Note

While still reviewing the caregiver study interview transcripts, I traveled to London to attend the 2017 Alzheimer's Association's International Conference. There, I found an amazing number of medical scientists, doctors, social scientists, and dementia industry professionals who had gathered—over 5,000 strong—to share, listen, and learn with colleagues as kindred spirits in a multifront research attack on this dreaded disease. I am hopeful my efforts will compliment theirs for making people the world over more aware of the current situation—and the need to eliminate the "silence" that too often shrouds afflicted individuals and affected families. If knowledge is indeed power—then information must be more openly shared by all those touched to build a broader understanding and more societal commitment to improve both treatment and caregiver resources.

What Are They Talking About?

An overriding lesson in the caregiver study participants' personal experiences was the importance of learning. Some read, others spoke to industry experts, and a few did neither. Overwhelmingly, those who sought to learn about what to expect, how to handle things, when and who to call for help, etc. went through their caregiver experience better. This book was designed to allow the caregivers themselves help educate whoever has taken an interest—just as they more readily accepted the advice from support groups than other sources. During my review of the interview transcripts, I found myself silently nodding (as though back in front of them) while hearing my own adage that had emerged, then stayed in my head: "If you care, become aware and then prepare."

> *"They're going to see signs of dementia. Things that they expect their parent to be able to do that they're not doing. Try to realize that they can't do it—even though they're going to try to convince you that they're fully capable of doing it, which is where the rub comes in. So you're balancing that in your head. They're trying to convince you they're still fully capable of doing this. You know that they always have been fully capable of doing this, and yet they're not getting it done. The checkbook's not balanced, or things are not happening the way they're supposed to happen…If you think they probably have dementia, treat them like they do—even though you don't have the proof yet…You need to watch out for them more than you probably think."[412]*

Many of the best solutions for preparing or dealing with becoming cognitively impaired or caregiving for such a family member were already spoken within the caregivers' words in "Love Thy Stranger." Additional caregivers' comments will be used for insights on items not mentioned or explained in the case stories.

A frequent notion within published Alzheimer's and caregiving papers, articles, books, organizational websites, as well as in conversations with scientists, doctors, academics, and industry professionals, has been how increasing public discussions and better awareness may move *Alzheimer's* from where *cancer* was a half century ago—back when cancer was far too frightening to be discussed.

To adequately inform on the experience of being a family caregiver, it is necessary to provide some basic understanding of their loved one's ailment(s). Much more can be learned from other books and websites pertaining to Alzheimer's, dementia, and other cognitive challenges. Among them, *The 36 Hour Day*, by Nancy L. Mace, MA, and Peter V. Rabins, MD, MPH,[413] has both medical and behavioral descriptions of the ailments and the issues they may create for both patient and caregiver. It has become a useful caregiver primer and is frequently suggested to people who find themselves taking on the caregiver role. The Alzheimer's Association[414] is the world's largest online subject content provider—with an expansive array of information, including their updated *Facts and Figures* and many other publications and resources for the general public. Their website also provides access to Alzheimer's awareness campaigns, research developments, support group locations, and other caregiver support items. The American Association of Retired Persons (AARP)'s research reports and other additional reference resources related to the various terms and items noted throughout this book are located in the *Notes* section.

Beyond those who have or will be mentioned, important research by pharmaceutical companies, neuroscientists, geneticists, sociologists, and others is ongoing and available in medical and industry journals or white papers.[415] Fascinating developments in the war on Alzheimer's and dementia are constantly available to those searching for them, such as the *Cedars-Sinai's* announcement of the possible use of high-definition retina scans for earlier detection of Alzheimer's,[416] or potential new brain imaging "biomarkers"[417] such as "Neurofilament light protein" (Nfl) in plasma for detecting and monitoring Huntington's disease.[418] There is no shortage of quality information available to those seeking it, and readers are encouraged to self-learn prior to becoming a caregiver or cognitively impaired.

Prior to my conducting this book's research study, I acquired over 30 years of industry experience professionally advising families on their personal financial and estate planning affairs. Family dynamics, investment availability, adequate insurance, and their care preferences were always critically important factors when they dealt with a long-term care illness—such as Alzheimer's or dementia. Even though none of my clients were invited to be included in my caregiver research study, lessons learned from the business world may provide a better understanding for some concerns identified by the case participants.

With due respect to others who may emphasize on some Alzheimer's, dementia, or caregivers' aspects in greater detail—this book will focus its effort to primarily provide readers better context for the items discussed by the caregiver study participants.

Types of Dementia

"There's all kinds of dementia—not just Alzheimer's. There's Lewy body—there's so many that attack the brain. If they could only find out what to do about it—how to ease the pain. If you watch them as they just—they just fall apart. To watch that day in and day out, it's…I'm sorry (crying)."[419]

It would likely be more confusing than helpful to attempt to list the more than 100 different types of dementia that have been identified. Those noted below are provided to demonstrate this point while reminding readers there are numerous resources to further study the medical conditions that could put someone into the family caregiver to a cognitively impaired person phenomenon studied in this book.

Table 1—(Adapted from *Managing Your Memory*)[420]

Major Types of Dementia

Alzheimer's disease - Pick's disease - frontotemporal dementia

vascular dementia (Lacunar state, Binswanger's disease) - Lewy body disease

Parkinson's dementia - supranuclear palsy - Huntington's disease

infections (general paresis - slow virus infections
- Creutzfeldt-Jakob disease)

hydrocephalus - demyelinating diseases - HIV
encephalopathy - semantic dementia

The varied causes on the many types of dementia continue to be researched with some inconsistencies for listing alcohol,[421] yet medications and head trauma can both mimic and lead to dementia.[422] Regardless of the cause or type of Alzheimer's or other dementia one may develop, their care levels and the available care choices are important to know.

> *"Well, it would be, you know—the toilet thing, the bath thing, the possibly feeding, walking—the whole gamut. I could do it maybe for a short time, but then I would be in the same position I think. And you hear that happening sometimes too. The caregiver gives too much. And no, 'They're not going into a facility. I'm going to hang onto them.' And they're the first ones to go because of the overwhelming stress and everything else. So, it's just a horrible disease. Hopefully, they'll find a cure one of these days. I've had the hope—not so much lately."*[423]

Care Levels

Activities of daily living,[424] or ADLs, are the primary drivers that determine the level of care needed for an Alzheimer's- or dementia-afflicted individual. They are considered the tasks necessary for taking care of one's self in everyday life, such as dressing, eating, bathing, transferring (moving from bed, chair, or commode), and toileting (or maintaining continence).[425] Mental incapacity or losing the ability to handle three or more of these basic ADLs most often are considered qualifying events for receiving care benefits from long-term care policies.

While insurance companies and medical care may still utilize the basic ADLs, the research study's family caregivers spoke of many problems or concerns outside of them. These are referred to as functional independence ADLs and include tasks necessary to maintain one's independence, such as handling one's checkbook, driving or using car services alone, doing laundry or cleaning, cooking, or getting groceries, etc.

Home health care agencies are frequently brought in when these functional independence ADLs become a concern, so individuals can sometimes remain longer in their homes or independent living apartments. Then, as their basic ADLs become compromised, other forms of home care are either added to the person's current dwelling, or they may need to be "placed" into a facility more suitable to their care needs.

> *"Some of them, they have to change the bed a couple of times a day—bathroom clean up and this sort of thing. One lady was saying that she was trying to give her husband a shower or something—he pooped on the floor in the shower. All kinds of the worst things that you can imagine that some of these people—I can't believe some of them are still hanging on and taking care of them."*[426]

Medical practitioners, continuing care facilities, long-term care insurance companies and caregivers also use ADLs to determine where the care should take place—or more specifically, where it may no longer be suitable for the ill person to live. Some of the greatest concerns voiced by the research study's family caregivers were *when* and *where* to properly care for their loved one.

Home Health Care

Home health care companies are usually hired in-home care aides, which provide non-nursing skill services in the home of the ill person. They are generally hired by the hour (most have a minimum number of hours per visit) to assist healthier single persons or to help home caregivers with tasks they cannot, or choose not to, do. A reoccurring comment by the caregivers was that many spouses do not enlist help early enough because they don't realize the compounding nature of the tasks they keep adding on—which becomes a problem for both spouses.

> *"You don't want to take care of yourself. You don't thing about—you just want to be there. You don't think about, 'Oh, so and so would be better at this than me.' You don't want anybody else to interfere with the way you're going to do it."*[427]

* * *

> *"When I started losing my patience, right toward the end and yelling at her rather than at the disease, I knew that I was in deep trouble at that point and something had to be done."*[428]

Assisted Living Facilities

Assisted Living Facilities, or ALFs, are usually senior-aged communities for individuals or couples in need of varying assistance with the basic activities of daily living mentioned previously. Although there are some small homes with only a few residents that could be placed into this category, most are apartment-style dwellings with common dining and activities areas. For individuals with mobility challenges, these communities often enable them greater socialization than they would have by themselves in a traditional house.

Health levels of the residents may vary greatly, with care plans being tailored to individuals' needs—and adjusted when warranted. Similar to home health care, non-nursing skilled assistance may be provided along with medication oversight or dispensing by some of the staff at the facility.

Sometimes ALF apartments may be attached or mixed within Independent Living Facilities—sharing the common areas, dining and activities. These "aging in place"–style communities can allow for friendships with neighbors to be maintained longer for individuals or couples, even as their lives become more restricted by a long-term care ailment. Caregiver support groups often hold meetings at ALFs, which simplifies attendance for the resident caregivers and may acquaint those still caregiving at home with the facility.

Because of the socialization and activities available at a well-run independent living or assisted living facility, these are often desired by those not wanting to be alone. The cost of these facilities ranges from one and a half times the rent of an area's non-senior apartment complexes to five or six times that amount—depending on amenities and demand. Affording these residences may be less formidable than first thought after realizing these moves generally entail leaving a private residence, which eliminates many home ownership expenses (e.g., insurance, property taxes, and maintenance) and allows the home to be sold to provide additional income toward the rent and care costs.

One way for family, friends, or their trusted advisors (e.g., doctors, financial advisors, lawyers, etc.) to help determine if a well spouse might benefit from relinquishing the chores of maintaining a house while being a caregiver would be to ask them: "Do you feel you own the house, or does the house own you?" Their answer should let them know if calling in more help or a move is worth considering.

Nursing Homes and Memory Care

Nursing facilities have private and semiprivate rooms similar to rehabilitation centers—which are sometimes available to serve other folks' temporary care needs. Memory care or "lockdown" facilities may also be multi-bed wards designed to protect their residents from themselves. Locking doors with passcodes for staff and visitors are used to keep those who might otherwise wander from becoming lost.

> *"Find the right facility first of all. There are poor skilled nursing centers. There are very good skilled nursing centers. There's a government website, I think it's under Medicare that rates nursing homes across the country."*[429]

For most, placement into a facility comes when all other options have been exhausted or are no longer feasible. The research study's caregivers who placed their loved ones seemed both relieved and guilty. The wives and daughters interviewed voiced more reluctance or anxiety over placing their loved ones into a facility when compared to the husbands and sons in the same study. However, there were exceptions to these majority feelings expressed in both gender segments.

> *"They're always going to be some problems but they're all very minor and they're taken care of... almost immediately. The staff are just so conscientious about what they're doing. The CNAs are remarkable, just remarkable. They treat those residents, including my wife, like family—I guess you might say, maybe even better."*[430]

Custodial care through end of life is provided in these facilities, and they are the most costly of the care options—unless compared to 24/7 care in a private residence. These facilities generally charge the most and are not mandated to accept Medicaid residents over those paying by insurance or out of pocket. As the wave of increased incidence for Alzheimer's and dementia approaches, a shortage of nursing home or memory ward beds would present additional challenges for millions of families. For those caregivers who will have to rely on Medicaid assistance because their loved one's health requires round-the-clock custodial care—it could be devastating.

> *"It's going to be necessary. You're going to have to make that decision—and there's no way in the world that you're going to be able to prevent that from happening. It's that simple, or complicated, whichever."*[431]

Family Affair

Researcher's Note

While I was sheltered as a child from my Mamaw's dementia, years later I simply became a busy young professional and distant stakeholder while my other grandmother was taking care of my grandfather who had Alzheimer's. She dutifully cared for him at home, but chose only to laugh and share with us grandchildren the "silly things" he would say or do.

She, herself, lived to 106 years old and was cognitively sharp to the end. In the 20 years following his passing, we often heard her laugh and say how Grandpa would wake up, forget who she was, and yell, "Hey, what are you doing here? You better get out before my wife comes in!" She also delighted in telling how after he'd been smoking for 70 years, she got him to stop.

Grandpa was rummaging through the kitchen drawers looking for matches. Grandma was worried about him burning down the house—so she asked, "What are you doing?" He said, "I'm looking for matches—I want to have a smoke." She calmly said, "You don't smoke anymore." He said, "I don't?" She said, "No, you gave that up a long time ago." Then she would smile, saying he just shrugged his shoulders and never smoked again.

While my grandmother was an extremely positive person, I now know that those years she spent as my grandfather's caregiver were not as jovial as she presented them to us. I loved my grandparents, yet since she never reached out—it never dawned on me to learn how he was really doing and if there were any ways I could have helped. Sometimes when you are a distant stakeholder, it is easy to miss opportunities to be more supportive. Embarrassingly, I found the old axiom "out of sight, out of mind" was very fitting.

Caregiver Selection

"I think that you should always be having conversations throughout your entire life about all of these things. My wife and I have had the conversation about what if one of us goes first? How we would deal with finances, which were in pretty good shape, and how we would go forward with different things if one of us were here alone." [432]

A majority of the family caregivers participants in this book's research study spoke of receiving little to no financial support from family, and only limited levels of emotional support from family—which were not as much as they may have wanted or needed. However, there was a significant minority of them who experienced quite positive emotional support and even some shared caregiving assistance within their families. The case stories' caregiver experiences and concerns were representational to some, but not all, of the more generalized expected responses noted by the study's industry professionals. Later, "Behind the Curtain" will discuss the research process and limitations a bit more. With already 5.5 million current caregivers to cognitively impaired family members, there is hope other family caregivers do (or will) experience greater support from children, siblings, or other relatives.

"What happens when Mom or Dad can't take care of themselves? What is the plan and can we save toward that plan? Can we have an understanding of which sibling is going to be the caregiver, so it doesn't just fall on the one who's closest or the one who has the most money? I think that that would really help families to continue to exist more as a family and not have so many disagreements and arguments and problems later…if there can be an understanding of who's going to do what." [433]

The academic research does show who is more likely within a family to become a caregiver based on large statistical caregiver surveys, but much of that data is not easily read by the public. This book is designed to help bridge the gap between practice and academia, so I will provide some of these researchers' findings where they relate to readers' concerns from the aforementioned expected wave of increased caregivers.

As with the previous family caregiver participant's comment, the study participants' information continues to reflect what may be found in the research. Caregiver selection is influenced by location and resources, as noted in this excerpt from a largely statistical report in the *Journal of Human Resources*:

> *"The ordered probit regression results confirm that factors like an adult child's sex, distance from parent, work status, and number of siblings are significant factors in decisions concerning how much care to provide for elderly parents."*[434]

Such articles chart the statistical prevalence for differing family relationships to become caregivers. It is sound science, but it is not written directly to a public audience, which could benefit from these many researchers' findings. This section will draw from that research but forgo the underlying mathematical equations of their studies. Instead, readers should compare their own family circumstances to the case stories presented, ahead of the coming increases in the number of family caregivers, to decide how they might best handle such an occurrence in the future.

Table 2

US Caregiver Statistics

- 60% / 40% = female caregivers vs. males
- 65% / 35% = female care recipients vs. males
- 0-20 / 20+ = lower weekly hour caregivers / higher weekly hour caregivers
- 24.4 = avg. number of hours caregiving weekly
- 44.6 = avg. number of hours spousal caregiving weekly
- 5x = how much more likely a child is to act as a caregiver to a parent or in-law than is a spouse
- 4x = the likelihood the caregiver is a spouse when the number of caregiving hours is high
- 4 years = average length of time caregiving
- 24% = caregivers for 5 or more years
- 2x = likelihood a higher hour caregiver's length is 10 or more years
- 48% = care recipients in private home

(Adapted from AARP's *Caregiving in the US* 2015)[435]

A family member's "desire" to keep their relative at home, their living "proximity" to the ill person, and their "perceived obligation" are the top three reasons for someone electing to act as a family caregiver.[436] This does not always mean that others within the family will have the same perspective as the family caregiver.

> *"Some people grow up without a strong sense*
> *of family or duty or honor.*
> *Some people grow up with that. I think that's*
> *a very individual thing."*[437]

* * *

> *"I had never been the one that was local, and*
> *I was always the one that was 'successful.' Right? I*
> *was the one that left and hasn't been around, so I*

think, I'm guessing resentment. Just this last year, my nephew got married and didn't invite us to the wedding. So, I think I got my answer on how they feel."[438]

Several of the research study participants were mystified by these differences in perspective within their families. Some had rebuffed offers for assistance and tried to handle everything themselves, while others never received or reached out for assistance. Whatever family dynamic may exist within a family, good or bad, family caregivers should realize that rather than do nothing and expect sudden changes in their long-standing relationships to take place without their direction—they can choose to build a support network themselves.

"It's still just me, because everybody's passed away. I have my husband and then I have my girlfriends and my church family, which is really more my family. They were all supportive. That was the support that I got from family. Sometimes family's not blood, I guess."[439]

Overall, the caregivers with families (or friends) maintaining higher levels of communication or assistance expressed less stressful experiences.

"If they're not taking care of themselves, they're eventually going to do that person, that loved one, no good."[440]

* * *

"They need a break. They just need a break, and if you're not able to come, are you able to pay for somebody else to be there for an hour once a month? Just give your sister a break. Pay for someone to come in for three hours so your sister can get out once a month."[441]

Family Discussion

There are many excellent advisors ready to assist individuals and families in all walks of professions. Doctors, nurses, lawyers, financial advisors, insurance agents, caregiver trainers, psychologists, and spiritual counselors may all figure prominently in the lives of those either preparing for, or already encountering, a cognitively impaired family member.

> *"Having the partnership between the attorney and the physician and open communication with the three of us, it was more bilateral. It wasn't like all three of us together on the phone, but it was bilateral with me as a pivot point in the middle and me having clear…authority was yeah, without question, you know, exceptionally valuable."*[442]

The specialized knowledge they possess in their respected fields means individuals seeking or requiring guidance do not have to become experts themselves. They merely need to establish contact with the appropriate ones as warranted. However, crucial for having these professionals effectively diagnose, analyze, or deduce what needs to be attended to—are the openness and honesty of the people who seek their guidance. It is imperative that you "help them, to help you."

Preparation, or the lack of it, in the areas of financial planning, legal documents, insurances, or family discussions can play pivotal roles in lessening or heightening the strife borne by the caregivers.

> *"Make sure that you've got…three main pieces in place…(1) A financial services planner person who can guide you through the bumps in the markets…(2) A strong relationship with some family attorney somewhere that knows the family, has talked to the principals and knows what they want and can step in and be the heavy so that you're not having to do that every day and…(3) That pri-*

mary care physician, having a relationship with that person, such that they're willing to get on the phone, that they'll do a speakerphone conference call exam—because not all doctors will do it."[443]

This book seeks to provide researcher's facts, practitioner's points, and caregivers' insights as advice for individuals to consider their own family situations. However, the general information discussed in this book should not in any way be misconstrued as providing personal legal, financial, insurance, or psychological recommendations—as such should be attended to directly with appropriately credentialed professionals.

Legal Documents

Having properly implemented legal documents (i.e., Durable Power of Attorney, Health Care Surrogate, Living Will, Will and/or Trust, etc.) already in order is imperative for families dealing with Alzheimer's or dementia. Once a person's ability to understand what they are signing is compromised, they are said to lack "legal capacity" and are no longer able to create new legal documents or update older ones. Legal documents sometimes needing to be created after an individual's incapacitation, other than merely updating a well-spouse's documents, can be far more complex—involving guardianships, if documents were not in proper order or special trusts as a part of Medicaid or Veteran's Administration benefit planning.

This book offers only a brief discussion on the importance of the various primary legal documents so that individuals and families may better discuss their personal needs with an attorney. Those seeking new legal documents must give clear direction to the attorney to ensure the documents, when prepared, will legally empower the people they wish to act on their incapacitation. The following form is provided to help readers, help the attorneys, to have others help them:

Family Fiduciary Checklist

Step 1: Think about it

Give thoughtful consideration for which individuals might best be selected to act upon one's incapacitation or death.

Step 2: Write it down

To establish clear direction of one's intended fiduciaries.

Step 3: Make it legal

Your list of desired primary, secondary, and subsequent fiduciaries (see form below) must be properly incorporated into wills, trusts, durable power of attorneys, and health surrogates.

Step 4: Talk about it

Let family or friends know who you have named to act as your fiduciaries ahead of a crisis. Give your trusted fiduciaries a copy of your legal documents and tell them where you will keep your originals.

Figure 1
Family Fiduciary Planning List

(Complete for *each* legal document to be prepared)

Primary Selection

Spouse A:_________________ Spouse B:_________________

Contingent Selection

Spouse A:_________________ Spouse B:_________________

Tertiary Selection

Spouse A:_________________ Spouse B_________________

The preceding table is a family fiduciary planning list for noting the desired persons to act upon one's incapacitation. This simple flowchart may be copied, filled out, and taken to an attorney who, by asking the party requesting the fiduciary updates to confirm them, can then attest they were given careful consideration by the signer—and thus be incorporated into new legal documents to ensure the desired persons will be empowered.

Durable Power of Attorney

For many family caregivers, this form is the most important document to have signed while their loved one still has legal capacity to name who they are choosing to act on their behalf in a wide variety of areas. Insurance, investment, and banking information are purposefully protected—especially for the elderly. For a family caregiver (other than one also titled on an account) to gain access to view holdings or be able to make necessary withdrawals or changes for the person needing care—a legal appointment is required. Having to file legal paperwork to become an incapacitated individual's appointed legal guardian can be avoided with a properly implemented Durable Power of Attorney.

> *"The first thing—is there anything legal? Like, who is power of attorney? All the legal issues need to be in place."*[444]

These documents grant a legal authority and a fiduciary duty[445] to whomever the signer has designated. (Recall the caregiver comment in "Love Thy Stranger" specifying it be a *durable* power of attorney.) His emphasis on that word is because the holder of a non-durable power of attorney ceases to have authority upon the issuer's incapacitation. The word *durable* means the person granting another to act on their behalf wishes it to continue even upon their incapacitation. State rules differ on these documents—including some which have allowed, then retracted, "springing" durable power of attorney documents that withheld legal authority until an incapacitation has occurred. Individuals desiring certain deferred fiduciary authority should meet with an estate/elder affairs attorney for solutions to their needs, to discuss such specific language within durable power of attorney documents or for successor trustees.

It is important to recognize that a durable power of attorney cannot legally command the named individual to act in that fiduciary role. The named person may have passed on, become health challenged or mentally incapacitated, or otherwise be unable or unwilling to act. Therefore, it is important to name a successor durable power of attorney and a third, or even fourth—with each in line and able to assume the role upon those prior to them withdrawing or becoming unavailable through death or incapacity.

All these issues should be discussed with the attorney drafting the durable power of attorney and again during periodic reviews for desired updates—especially after a person relocates to another state, which may require updates or replacement of legal documents because of variances within the state laws.

Health Care Surrogate

Whether these documents are called health care surrogate, health care power of appointment, or some other version—their purpose is to name the individual entrusted with legally speaking on one's behalf for medical decisions. Health Information Privacy Protection Act (HIPPA)[446] rules can cause frustrations for family caregivers at not being immediately granted health information on a loved one until they can show they have a right to know or speak on behalf of their family member.

It is wise for caregivers to always keep copies of health care surrogate/appointment/proxy documents readily available (as well as their relatives' other documents putting them into a position of authority).

*"If the parents refuse or don't fill out the forms
to give you the authority for HIPPA and for financial power and things like that 'cause they're wor-*

ried and scared about what you're going to do, then you've got an underlying problem that's going to be there that is really hard to manage."[447]

As with the durable power of attorney—there should be successive or contingent parties named to act within a health care surrogate/appointment/proxy document. When there is a difference between who is named as a durable power of attorney versus the health care surrogate/agent/proxy, the health decisions are generally made by this fiduciary's direction ahead of the wishes of the non-health care fiduciary.

Living Wills/DNRs

Loving one's family sometimes means helping to ease their burden and/or pain. Few areas underscore this more than having a living will already in place ahead of a medical catastrophe. Allowing others to know one's wishes significantly aids caregivers in dealing with the end-of-life issues.

"Unfortunately, when someone does start to have Alzheimer's, they're unable to communicate verbally, necessarily what their wishes are. So if all of that is written down, what a relief to the caregiver because he had his living will…As the person advocating for him, I already knew what his wishes were. I didn't have to question if I was doing the right thing when it came to pull the feeding tube and take the ventilator out. I didn't have to bear the burden of like, 'Did I do the right thing?'"[448]

Living wills document one's wishes for continuance of care or removal of care upon certain conditions. This helps family caregivers to respectfully carry out their loved one's instructions instead of being placed into the unsettling position of having to make the decision when to end feeding, oxygen, ventilation, or other life-support machines. There are also times when a family member may be in denial or in disagreement with the ill person's own wishes for not wanting to prolong their life. A well-drafted living will may help to have one's own wishes be carried out—while freeing caregivers from making end-of-life decisions. Guilt was a reoccurring theme within the caregiver study participants' comments.

> *"Absolutely doing a living will and then the financial planning. Get that house in order so that that person's wishes are very clear…that is the touchstone that removes all of the arguments…If it's clear what Mom or Dad wants and they've said, 'This is what I want,' and it's written and it's signed…you can pull that back out and say, 'We're doing things because this is what they said they wanted to do.' That trumps all of that, 'Well, I think this is best,' or 'I think that's best'…I think that's huge."*[449]

DNRs, or "do not resuscitate" forms, are commonly placed on file by hospitals, nursing homes, memory care units, or assisted living facilities and may be kept visually accessible in private homes. Without documented proof that an individual (or their health care surrogate/agent/proxy) has stated "not" to render medical attention, such as cardiopulmonary resuscitation, emergency responders may be obligated to do so—even if it is unwanted.

Wills and Trusts

Alongside durable power of attorney and health care surrogate/ appointment/proxy documents used to grant authority to others in the event of an incapacitation, may be successor trustee provisions. Assets titled in trust's name will be accessed or utilized for care at the direction of whomever the original trustee (or grantor) may have pre-named. An Alzheimer's- or dementia-afflicted individual with a trust would have acting trustees or successor trustees use their fiduciary authority in utilizing the trust assets on behalf of that incapacitated person in accordance to the document's directions during their lifetime. Upon that individual's death, the empowered trustee(s) would distribute their trust assets in accordance to the trust distribution schedule.

On a will, the person named to act as executor/executrix/personal representative does not hold any authority over the ill individual's assets during their lifetime. Instead, empowerment under the document begins when the person has died. The responsibility of the executor/executrix/personal representative is to then settle the person's affairs, much like the trustee above, in accordance to the will's stated provisions for bequests and/or amount of estate share to be received. The person's passing also ends the legal authority (or ability to act further) as a named durable power of attorney.

> *"I did not get all of the taxes filed accurately and on time. I did not get the estate settled in a timely manner, and in fact, the estate has not been settled…I've now stepped aside…and allowed my brother to become executor of the estate."*[450]

A few of the study's family caregivers expressed exhaustion after their loved one had passed and looked upon settling the estate as a chore, sometimes delaying or prolonging their grieving. To help them, individuals should complete their trust's "tangible list of personal property" or their will's "separate writing." These lists (typically created, signed, and dated at home after the documents have been signed with the attorney) allow an individual to also give their trustee or executor/executrix/personal representative direction for handing out their personal possessions. (Remember the heartache expressed by one of the case study participants at her siblings' differing regard for their mother's belongings.) Providing some direction by writing down the items important to be placed with heirs can help simplify estate settlements and minimize emotional conflicts.

It is important to clarify desired scope of authority for these fiduciaries with an attorney prior to the documents' drafting or updating to avoid conflicts when differing family members have been simultaneously named with different authorities. Such as one child listed as the durable power of attorney, another as the first successor trustee, and possibly a third as the health care surrogate/agent/proxy.

Without practicing law, most financial planners encourage their clients not to do this. Instead, uniformly appointing the same order of primary, contingent, and tertiary fiduciaries usually allows for fewer family disagreements. "Co-anything" is frequently not found by the cofiduciaries to be the intended "fairest" way to avoid naming one over another or having them "share the load." Having to coordinate signatures and/or decisions for important caregiving, financial, or medical issues can be logistically and emotionally challenging. Attorneys do sometimes draft coinciding authorities, in which each can act independently of the other, but even this arrangement works well only where high family harmony exists.

Operation of Law

Some assets are not passed on by wills or trusts, but instead, are passed on by operation of law. These properties or accounts bypass the probate or trust administration process with a legal transfer of ownership taking place upon a person's passing because they were jointly titled with someone else or there were named heirs on file. Life insurance policies, IRAs, and annuities list the intended heirs as beneficiaries, whereas brokerage accounts, mutual fund companies, and stock transfer agents use "Transfer on Death" (TOD) forms to list the heirs. Banks and credit unions use "In Trust For" (ITF) or "Payable on Death" (POD) forms to do the same.

Many of these accounts or investments may be jointly titled, such as, Joint Tenants with Right of Survivorship (JTWROS), which automatically grants the survivor full title. Properties, investments, or accounts solely in the name of an owner, without named heirs, will be assumed as intended to be handed out in accordance with the decedent's estate disposition—which means they should follow the directions of the decedent's will, or trust, if they had a "pour over will," through probate or trust administration.

Without a will, trust, or operation of law transfer, these assets would be subject to the decedent's own state's rules of "intestacy"—which can be a far more cumbersome and costly task for the family settling the estate. (Remember the frustration voiced by the caregiver in "Love Thy Stranger" whose brother failed to have their parent name beneficiaries or have the wills updated.)

When operation of law methods are used, it is important to realize that these forms are also unable to be updated by an incapacitated individual or changed by their legal fiduciaries. Ensuring these forms name one's desired heir(s) properly should be a part of each family's financial and legal preparation routine and should be periodically reviewed and adjusted as warranted.

Elder Financial Exploitation

The looming wave of baby boomer cognitive impairment could bring with it another unfortunate consequence—the propensity for a similar increase in Elder Financial Exploitation. The vulnerabilities of those with Alzheimer's or dementia are undeniable. Having over $10 trillion of wealth by 2050 to be controlled by those without legal capacity should greatly heighten the concern over this problem.[451] The National Center on Elder Abuse defines *financial exploitation* as "the illegal taking, misuse, or concealment of funds, property, or assets of a vulnerable elder."[452] Long before the caregiving begins, individuals developing Alzheimer's or other dementias can become easy targets for those intent on taking advantage of their growing confusion.

> *"The neighbors were making their accusations about us trying to put her away, blah, blah, blah, whatever…and I had to get on the phone with the bank this particular day. She's like, 'Here, you tell her, Honey, what I want to do.'*
>
> *I went on the phone with the bank and the girl at the bank, she says, 'Since I have permission to talk to you,' she said, 'I was hoping I would see you*

or something'…She said, 'Your grandmother comes to the bank every single week and withdraws $500 cash.'

So, I was like, 'Oh my gosh'…I said, 'Does she come in the front door…or is she coming in the side?' She goes…'That's just it. It's not on the camera. We've even looked to see who was bringing her because we've been curious ourselves,' and…'We don't know. She comes up the steps.'

I was just livid. I thought to myself, 'Here she is with a cane, very unsteady, has already had multiple falls at home, never broke a bone, thank God, and somebody's sending her up the steps in the bank.'

I'm pretty sure it was the neighbor. That may be why they didn't want her put away."[453]

Perhaps even more disturbing is that 90% of elder abuse cases involves a family member.[454] Consider the following comments—first, by Kathleen Quinn (Executive Director of the National Adult Protective Services Association to the US Senate Special Committee on Aging), then, by two of the research study participants when they took over as caregivers in their families:

"Sadly, and too many—shockingly, the vast majority…of reported elder abuse is committed by the older victim's own family: adult children, grandchildren, nieces and nephews and sometimes siblings."[455]

* * *

"My mom was basically treated like a bank, only it was all withdrawals."[456]

* * *

> *"If it would go through Medicare instead of having the 'spend-down' and everything—so that they can qualify for Medicaid to get any type of companion services—I think that the rate of neglect would go down. Exploitation…I've seen good people turn bad because of caregiver stress…I saw what the opportunity gave to one of my family members that was able to take advantage completely of the finances."*[457]

During my 25 years of experience as a Certified Financial Planner™ Professional working with seniors and their financial affairs, I developed a heightened concern and awareness of elder vulnerabilities. The overwhelming majority of family caregivers are earnest fiduciaries who would not think of misusing their role for financial exploitation. Unfortunately, there is still a very small percentage of these family members who do.

I consider these people part of a group I have labeled Inappropriate Family Fiduciaries, or IFFs. The 2018 Senior Safe Act[458] provides "whistle-blower" protections to financial institutions who suspect an elder may be unduly influenced by someone or who may have empowered an IFF.

Presently, there are many industry guidelines for voluntary reporting of suspicious behavior, but regulators should also keep in mind the plight of the trustworthy caregivers. They may better constrain future elder exploitation by increasing mandatory training in the financial services and other elder-engaged industries to be alert for exploitation warning signs, then providing civil protections for those reporting their suspicions.

The alternative of enacting a broad scope of mandatory reporting for all unusual elder/family member financial transactions could be quite hurtful to large numbers of honest caregivers and be less effective at controlling the problem.

Imagine if all elementary school teachers were "required" to file a suspicious injury report to the Division of Child Services whenever a child came in off the playground sporting a new bruise. Parents would be outraged and insulted, if all were visited by an investigator—even though there is a small possibility that the teacher could have seen a possible abuse case. Just as we want our teachers to be aware, ask questions, then report suspicious issues to a superior—so should we ask elders to be monitored by those in position to notice elder exploitation.

Train them and expand personal whistle-blower protections, but do not mandate too broad a spectrum of circumstances requiring reports—only to waste investigators' resources, while insulting and upsetting the millions upon millions of earnest family caregivers.

Still, as an advocate to combat Elder Financial Exploitation and Abuse by that small percent of unscrupulous family members, I did have an opportunity to present a 17-year longitudinal case study, *Failure to Avert an Inappropriate Family Fiduciary,* in a webcast to a group within the Financial Planning Association in March of 2017.[459]

The case centered on the consequences of not discussing who within a person's family (i.e., children, grandchildren, nephews, nieces, etc.) were capable and could be trusted to always act in one's best interest should they become incapacitated—and who might not. I told the attending educators and advisors that personal financial planners needed to:

> *"Shake the family tree…because while most*
> *trees bear fruit, some are full of nuts—and you need*
> *to know!"*[460]

My point was relatives are routinely listed in legal documents by birth order or proximity, rather than careful consideration of the financial and/or medical decision responsibilities the documents would empower these family fiduciaries to handle. Additionally, this same consideration must be given to "who else" would be a good selection for the role—as their first-named choice may predecease, be physically or mentally unable, or simply be unwilling to act for them.

Most spousal caregivers in the study admitted their named durable power of attorney was their Alzheimer's- or dementia-stricken spouse—which could have been a problem if left unchanged.

"As a matter of fact, we talked about that when she was well. The expectation's…the man dies sooner, gets ill sooner and the wife has the burden. That's kind of how we were thinking—but, it didn't work out that way."[461]

It is wise to always name a backup person to the contingent in case of multiple family illnesses or deaths—which occurred in the aforementioned webcast case. Sadly, that case underscored that the further down the family tree one names potential fiduciaries, the greater the likelihood the advisors may be unfamiliar with their character or abilities.

So it is vital for all individuals to think carefully about their fiduciary selections, while they still have their legal capacity, then have an attorney incorporate their preferred order of succession within their legal documents.

While waiting for regulatory improvements to protect future elders caught up in the wave of baby boomer cognitive impairment, there are steps individuals can take to safeguard against falling prey to an IFF themselves.

The *Four I's of IFF Empowerment* slide, from the aforementioned webcast presentation, has been included as Figure 2—to help guide individuals and families to avoid the unintentional empowerment of an inappropriate family fiduciary.

Figure 2

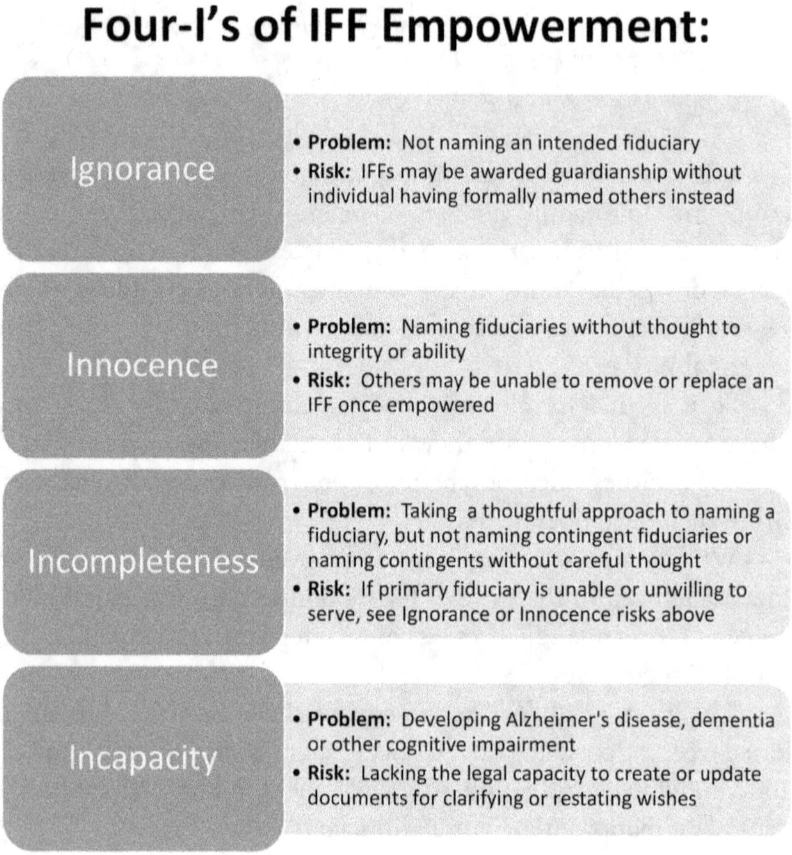

Four-I's of IFF Empowerment:

Ignorance
- **Problem:** Not naming an intended fiduciary
- **Risk:** IFFs may be awarded guardianship without individual having formally named others instead

Innocence
- **Problem:** Naming fiduciaries without thought to integrity or ability
- **Risk:** Others may be unable to remove or replace an IFF once empowered

Incompleteness
- **Problem:** Taking a thoughtful approach to naming a fiduciary, but not naming contingent fiduciaries or naming contingents without careful thought
- **Risk:** If primary fiduciary is unable or unwilling to serve, see Ignorance or Innocence risks above

Incapacity
- **Problem:** Developing Alzheimer's disease, dementia or other cognitive impairment
- **Risk:** Lacking the legal capacity to create or update documents for clarifying or restating wishes

(Tiller, *Failure to Avert an Inappropriate Family Fiduciary*, 2017)

Money Matters

Long-Term Care Planning

Researcher's Note

My most eye-opening experiences with Alzheimer's came by way of my professional vocation as a Certified Financial Planner™ Practitioner. In a career where people openly share their hopes, dreams, fears, joys, and sorrows—I learned the oversights of my youth as I counseled many families through their own Alzheimer's and dementia journeys. Afterward, the family caregivers often expressed great appreciation for my calm presence, concerned advice, and personal encouragement. Financially, some were better prepared for their challenges, others not as much—but like most financial advisors, I tried to help them make the best decisions they could with what they had. Ironically, although I was several stakeholder layers outside from where I had been for my grandparents, these Alzheimer's encounters touched me more—albeit still as an indirect stakeholder. I have spent many years encouraging clients and other advisors to learn how to better prepare or deal with a cognitively impaired family member. This book is an extension of that effort, with an intent to engage a broader audience to discuss these issues so that many others may be helped.

* * *

In "Love Thy Stranger," financial concerns or strains families often contend with were not demonstrated alongside the other Alzheimer's and dementia caregiver issues. My case research has attempted to provide a relatable understanding of this growing caregiver phenomenon, but it is only a partial explanation. Many areas deserving discussion did not emerge from the particular research sample studied. Some of the reasons for those limitations will be discussed in "Behind the Curtain."

The research study's industry professionals interviewed affirmed the existing literature that the cost of care remains an enormous and typically undiscussed hurdle for individuals, families, and even governments. Individuals' or families' resources and Medicaid are the "two major payers" for nursing homes—the larger payer being

Medicaid.[462] *Forgotten Faces: Family Caregiver Voices'* study sample was a near inversion to the general population for Medicaid filings. Other research has shown "one-fifth" of nursing home bills are borne by families "at a considerable financial burden."[463]

Readers should keep in mind that an added burden of financial challenges can greatly exacerbate whatever problems the caregiver(s) will encounter.

> *"I looked into, possibly, divorce, because I thought, 'Well, divorce, I can at least keep half of it.' I didn't go that route, but I looked into that. It was more for my own financial security as I got older, because I know that it can devastate whatever you do have… 'What can I do to take care of him for as long as he lives, but also keep some of it for me because… I'm getting older. I'm going to need some care too."*[464]

As a researcher, I followed the disciplined scientific methods for gathering data from a *sample population* of caregivers. There will be millions of people caught up in the coming wave of cognitively impaired family members needing care. While the experiences of the 24 individuals in the study may resonate with most readers, they do not reflect all of the caregiver circumstances or concerns others may face. Most caregiver subjects' commentaries represented in "Love Thy Stranger" spoke of having been financially able to handle the costs of care for their cognitively impaired family member. Some merely spent as was needed from their loved one's accumulated investments, while others had long-term care insurance benefits available to minimize the investment asset depletion. Unfortunately, there were also several study participants, whose comments were not reflected in the book's case stories, without either insurance or adequate financial resources available.

The coming increase of millions upon millions more of cognitively impaired family members needing long-term care demands everyone's attention. One of the objectives for this book on the caregiver phenomenon is to encourage a more open discussion between families, professionals, and policymakers. This was also the sentiment of the brief working paper I withdrew from the 2017 CFP Board's Academic Colloquium, *Medicaid Millionaires: The Ethics of Evasion,*[465] restated here:

> "The aging of the baby boomers brings with it a tremendous increase in the nation's long-term care need, with no current agreement on who should pay the cost. Societal ethical boundaries, moral opinion and individuals' willingness to financially participate in: higher taxes, mandated long-term care insurances or family responsibilities toward the long-term care costs—should be surveyed, studied and acted upon by policymakers without delay."[466]

As a practitioner-scholar, I continue to share the perspective of many financial planners and/or insurance professionals who encourage their clients to be adequately protected from the unknown. These advisors are sometimes frustrated that more people do not better prepare themselves ahead of potential problems. Most individuals who are intent on securing themselves or their families do use insurances, but sometimes they leave protection gaps, which could make them vulnerable in certain circumstances:

Figure 3

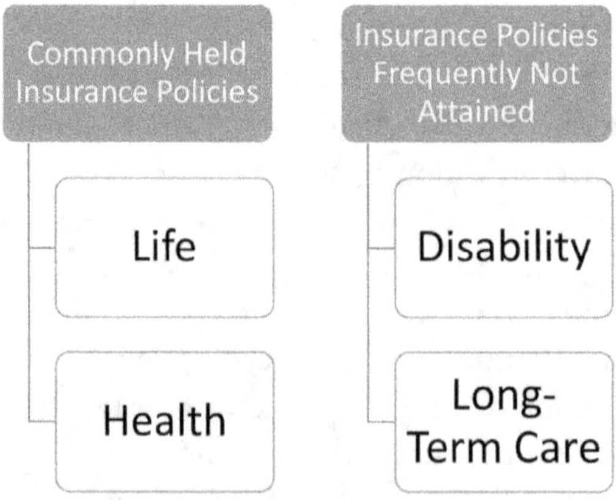

For a few people, the unattained supplementary protection policies are unavailable to them because of locale or current health status. Others avoid them because the circumstances being insured against are too disconcerting to discuss, while still more are concerned over the cost of coverage as an additional expense. Both reasons are understandable, but advisors know individuals forgoing broader protections may result in significant or even tragic consequences for some of them.

"He didn't even want to discuss it. Absolutely no way did he want to discuss it."[467]

Sadly, this caregiver's comment was on her husband's refusal of their financial advisor's recommendation of long-term care (LTC) insurance—only a few years before he was diagnosed with Alzheimer's.

Imagine if automobiles were sold with customers having to "add on" seat belts and airbags as options. Would these same consumer purchasing behaviors exist? I hope not; otherwise, many folks would opt out—either not wishing to think about the possibility of sustaining an injury or death in their new vehicle, or simply choosing to "save the money and take their chances."

People sometimes choose to "self-insure"—meaning they will set aside reserves or earmark resources to be utilized for a lengthy period of care. Others opt to transfer the risk of having to afford such care to an insurance company by purchasing an LTC policy. Many more have simply not made any plans or provisions for addressing the possibility of a long-term illness.

Self-insurers with adequate assets still warrant discussions with advisors and family on prioritization of spend-down and care preferences. Having appropriate family fiduciaries already properly named within one's legal documents is also important—to first ensure funds for care are readily available to the fiduciary, and then to keep those assets from becoming an elder financial exploitation temptation.

"I'm trying to come up with $4,500 a month to pay his bills. Plus, you know…living expenses.

*Thank goodness we had the investments, and the
insurances and things that were available.*[468]

Yet even those with significant assets sometimes choose to obtain long-term care coverage to lessen the spend-down of other assets being used by a spouse for income or earmarked for certain legacy objectives. Regardless of an intended insured's available financial resources or motivations for seeking LTC coverage, there are several types of policies available. Each of these may have a variety of benefit variations, confusing insurance language and complicated clauses.

Rather than view them as complex contracts to be avoided, those seeking good insurance coverage should realize their first step is to seek a good insurance agent. Many insurance agents and financial advisors offer LTC policies. A good agent will be licensed in the intended insured's state, knowledgeable about the different policies available, and get to know the individual's or couple's preferences, needs, and financial abilities—before making a recommendation.

LTC Insurance 101

Some LTC policies are designed to provide a benefit for a limited time frame, others provide lifetime coverage. Coverage is often selected based upon the amount of available benefits per day, month, or total under the contract. LTC policies pay benefits upon an insured's inability to perform certain activities of daily living, or becoming cognitively impaired. Some may reimburse the insured for qualifying expenses incurred, while others may directly pay the health providers.

The amount of available benefit may be static or different depending upon the location for care—such as home care, assisted living facilities, nursing, or memory care. To become insured, there is typically a medical underwriting—with younger and healthier individuals seeking coverage paying lower premiums and older or less healthy individuals paying more—or possibly being declined. Assuming a person is medically able, an ideal policy should match the insured's desired coverage, be within his/her financial ability to afford, and be kept in force through time of potential claim.

Regulations designed to protect the public from an insurance company becoming insolvent have historically performed well compared with other areas of financial industry protections. However, this does not mean that once an LTC policy is obtained, it will remain in force until needed. Some LTC policies function as a two-party agreement for coverage (i.e., the insured and the insurer) with both parties necessary for its continuance. Think of car insurance or homeowners' insurance for a moment. If policyholders continue to pay their premiums, the company continues to provide insurance coverage.

Insurance companies keep track of their "lapse rate"—which is the amount of policies that are discontinued by the insureds. LTC policies have a low lapse rate—as those seeking it are more apt to keep it because their concerns for needing the coverage generally do not diminish as they age.

To safeguard against an insurance company raising premiums to encourage more policyholders to lapse their coverage, agents may recommend policies with fixed premiums at companies with long histories of resisting rate hikes. LTC policies with fixed premiums generally cannot be increased without the company seeking approval from a state insurance commissioner's office. If a requested rate increase is not granted, the insurer has the right to discontinue offering coverage in that state. This could pose a problem for a now uninsured person if such an occurrence happened after becoming too old or ill to acquire alternative LTC coverage elsewhere.

Those who want even greater assurance their future coverage will remain in place can seek either "paid up" LTC policies or "linked-benefit" polices—which are actually life insurance policies designed to provide a significantly higher LTC benefit than the death benefit. Depending upon one's state of residence, these types of policies may be available in single-premium or multiple-year premiums. These policies may include inflationary riders to increase the benefit base over time. Some may even offer a partial or full return of premium—although most advisors would be hesitant to recommend their clients allow them to lapse.

Couples sometimes pursue long-term care insurance for emotional, not just financial, reasons. Having a "peace-of-mind" LTC policy may help combat a spouse's common instinct to do all the caregiving without assistance. This concept can be very effective because, generally, the only way to utilize an LTC policy benefit is to have outside professional help enlisted in the care—and few people would allow an insurance company to be "off the hook" by ignoring benefit funds once available.

Available resources for self-insuring, health challenges for underwriting and budgeting for premiums may all remain factors for consideration or obtaining LTC insurance. Those wanting to learn more about what coverage is available for them and how it might fit into their planning should remember: The key to getting good coverage lies in first speaking with a good insurance agent—and there are plenty to be found.

Researcher's Note

I have used this last LTC insurance concept in case either my wife or I fall prey to Alzheimer's or other ailments. The goal being to transfer some of the financial risk and lower the emotional toll for the well spouse.

Over time, these benefits will have greatly compounded with the inflationary riders, and the policies cannot be revoked by the insurer (or even a successor entity). The available funds should help protect myself or my wife from becoming overwhelmed by the physical caregiving tasks should either of us be incapacitated.

Our objective is for either of us to still be there, but to "supervise" as much of the caregiving tasks as possible, rather than "doing" all the physical caregiving ourselves. Because we've selected "linked-benefit" policies, if we are fortunate enough not to use the LTC benefits for home care, assisted living, nursing or memory care—the policies will not have been "wasted premiums" because then they will pay a life insurance death benefit to the survivor or our heirs.

Another peace-of-mind value is if the surviving spouse becomes incapacitated, our contingent family fiduciary will be less burdened by being able to use the LTC policy's benefits to hire outside help or for a move into a suitable care facility.

Because our policies also have return of premium features—which offer a provocative sum at the expense of forfeiting our appreciated LTC benefits—I periodically remind my wife, "They wouldn't offer it unless they wanted us to take it." Then I say, "Never, never, never let the insurance company 'off the hook' on our LTC policies."

Medicare, Medicaid, and VA Benefits

There is an important issue needing recognition in this book. The caregiver research study sample's case stories are nearly an inverse percentage on Medicaid filings versus occurrences within the general population.

> *"I had gone to a lawyer to see about Medicaid.*
> *I never got to that point, but I was in the process of*
> *seeing what I could do. We don't have a fortune, but*
> *seeing what we could do to—I guess the term would*
> *be to shelter money…I mean, a loved one probably*
> *should be placed, but financially, it's devastating to*
> *the family."[469]*

Medicare is a federal health program for people 65 years or older and is sometimes confused with Medicaid. Medicare and Medicaid both grew out of the Social Security program in 1965. Medicaid is a state-administered federal/state cooperative program to provide medical assistance to those without resources.[470] Another researcher characterized Medicaid as a "needs-based program" and Medicare as an "entitlement program."[471] It is not unusual for people to become confused between Medicare and Medicaid, as both programs cover health challenges for seniors. However, they cover different health items, are administered at different governmental levels, and have very different areas of coverage. A local caregiver support group charitable organization's retired director once told me part of this confusion is because of people's common "misconception" that custodial care needs for individuals with Alzheimer's or dementia patients are covered by Medicare.[472] Medicaid is the program turned to by families of individuals with Alzheimer's or dementia that provides many long-term care benefits generally excluded from Medicare's coverage.

Medicaid addresses these needs for those who qualify, but coverage rules differ state to state. Although there are some variances on the amount of long-term care or nursing costs paid for by individuals or families, there is no dispute that Medicaid has become the largest "payer" or "funding source" of long-term care costs in the nation[473] and, as such, requires some discussion and caregiver commentary.

Figure 4

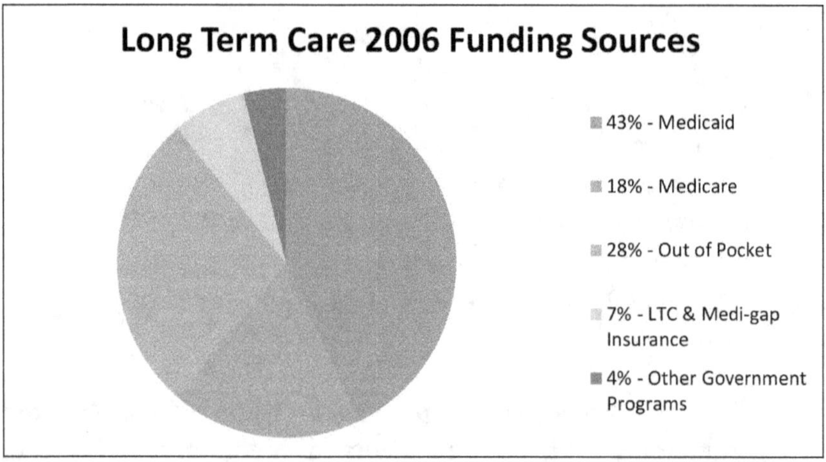

Long Term Care 2006 Funding Sources

43% - Medicaid

18% - Medicare

28% - Out of Pocket

7% - LTC & Medi-gap Insurance

4% - Other Government Programs

(Adapted from Avalere Health Data, 2008)[474]

Medicaid and the Veterans Administration's (VA) Aid and Attendance program both may provide some resources toward long-term care for those without adequate resources who qualify. These programs' asset and income-based qualifying systems often seem similar, but have significant differences, which should be known before applying for either.

For Medicaid, each state has its own rules on the amount of income, "countable or excluded assets," "look-back" rules, etc. These items are best discussed with a properly credentialed advisor—such as an experienced Elder Affairs Attorney. The VA's Aid and Attendance qualifications may also merit consulting an attorney because of the potential for one benefit's qualifying method to disqualify an individual for the other.

There are important state differences for qualifying for Medicaid assistance, although common to most is that benefits are only made available to pay for the care of individuals with less than $2,000 of countable assets and a limited monthly income level.

> *"The time is coming when I can get on Medicaid. I sold my house up North. I just sold it last week or two weeks ago, and that money will help out. They say if I get my money down low enough, they can help me get on Medicaid. I'm not to that point yet."*[475]

The history of Medicaid qualifying rules is long and varied, with both sides of the asset transfer debate offering strong arguments for the perspectives they hold. I have long argued, "Before the baby boomers' LTC needs 'Bust the Medicaid Trust,' an exploration on the ethics in avoiding Medicaid's spend-down provisions is warranted."[476] Some argue it is a needs-based program designed to help the "impoverished,"[477] citing the laws not being enforced were written to prohibit purposeful impoverishment to qualify.[478] Others ask why Medicare will pay for major illnesses but not long-term care, thereby causing some to feel they simply were "hit with the wrong disease."[479]

> *"'The first thing you got to do…is get him Medicaid qualified,' or whatever they call it. She said, 'Because it's a five-year look back.' That's what I did. I immediately made an appointment with the attorney and went down and talked to him and moved the money around so that I wouldn't be*

> *broke…I would have been left with probably very*
> *little, by the time you take care of them and pay for*
> *their medical and all that.*"[480]

Families sometimes seek to transfer assets out of the ill spouse's name to help them qualify. However, there are rules governing the allowable limits and timetables for doing so. Failure to adhere to the Medicaid "spend-down" rules can result in significant delays for receiving assistance or disqualification. Most financial and legal professionals welcome using available asset transfer rules to protect a well spouse from becoming impoverished by their ill spouse's care costs. However, some believe these transfer rules can be used too liberally by wealthy families whereby non-spouse relatives avoid spending down the ill person's available assets to maintain their inheritance.

Still others assert that forcing those who did save must spend down their own assets, while providing benefits to those who did not prepare is akin to the "ant and the grasshopper" fable. Who is right? Who is wrong? That answer differs, depending on circumstances and perspectives. As a researcher, a practitioner, and an elder advocate—I welcome this topic to become a public discussion ahead of the impending increase of individuals who will become cognitively impaired as the baby boomers age.

> *"I stopped working to take care of him; there-*
> *fore, my Social Security is less which is totally*
> *unfair. I worked 45 years and I worked hard. And*
> *just because it would have cost us more for me to go*
> *to work and get the Social Security.*"[481]

None of the caregiver participants in the research study spoke at length about VA benefits. However, as a practitioner-scholar, I am familiar with the "nonlegal advice" basic explanation likely to be offered by a Certified Financial Planner™ Practitioner ahead of a client's further investigation of whether or not to pursue VA Aid and Attendance benefits.[482]

The VA's Aid and Attendance benefits are sometimes touted as a long-term care resource "already earned" by a veteran or a veteran's surviving spouse that may assist with home care, assisted living, or even nursing home costs.

> *"Don't be a victim: Be aware of pension poaching scams."*
>
> (US Veterans Administration
> Postcard Warning)[483]

Like Medicaid, there is now a "look-back" on transferred assets to qualify, so beware of advisors who recommend doing so to immediately lower both asset and income levels. The VA's website cautions families against various scams designed to "qualify" individuals for these benefits. They have termed these as "pension poaching scams." Some may charge outrageously inappropriate fees for their services, while still others may offer "no cost" advice—not disclosing their payments from the investment or insurance mechanisms utilized to effect such transfers.

There are both reputable and nonreputable companies seeking to advise families on qualifying for these benefits. (See the VA's warning note inserted above.) Sometimes this strategy is pursued by the families with these advisors or on their own without having fully considered a cognitively impaired person's longer-term needs. This will sometimes upset lawyers and financial planners because some recommended strategies to qualify for VA benefits will also undermine an ability to qualify for Medicaid.

The rules governing both of these programs are complex, so this book cannot offer qualifying advice to individuals or families. Therefore, anyone seeking to attain either VA or Medicaid benefits should obtain qualified counsel (perhaps even an attorney in the ill-person's state-of-care residence with a board certification in Elder Law) before making any gifts, transfers, or other asset changes.

Researcher's Note

Those seeking benefits would be wise to heed the VA's warnings. Medicaid planning or VA benefit planning done incorrectly could result in significant costs and/or disqualifications for families.

Defining the appropriateness to individuals or policymakers on qualifying levels or transfer rules for either Medicaid or Veterans Benefits is beyond this book's objectives. However, the sustainability of these programs may depend upon a public discussion ahead of the anticipated increase in families that may need their assistance.

Policymakers may make significant changes to these and other programs that individuals should be aware of and incorporate into their own families' long-term care planning. Current state eligibility differences for assistance versus creating a national standard may not be possible with Medicaid, not Medicare, currently being the nation's primary payer of long-term care. Ahead of policy changes, further research should be undertaken at the state and federal levels on population demographic shifts and the potential budget impacts of the aging baby boomers' long-term care needs.

Longevity and Morbidity Baby Boomer Retirement Risks

In the financial industry, discussions of risk often center on the possibility of loss. People are generally already aware of the risk-reward relationship for investing—that to attain a potentially greater return, an investor must also be willing to sustain a greater possibility of loss. Naturally, it is important for retirees to guard against loss of their resources from unsuccessful investments or becoming a victim of Elder Financial Exploitation. However, there are additional "retirement risks" that should be recognized to prepare for them properly. Longevity Risk is simply the possibility of outliving one's resources. A significant factor directly affecting Longevity Risk is Inflation Risk—the possibility of costs rising over time—which could deplete resources sooner than expected.

"Financial is a big, big, big, big issue because they can live for years."[484]

An important but often overlooked retirement risk item is Morbidity Risk—the possibility of suffering an illness or injury that will require financial resources. Potential Alzheimer's, dementia, and other long-term cognitive illnesses discussed in this book would all be considered Morbidity Risks for retirees. Longevity, itself, is a factor for increasing Morbidity Risk because the incidence of Alzheimer's or dementia increases with age—affecting approximately one out of every three 85-year-olds.[485]

> *"If he lives as long as his mother did…I do keep that in the back of my mind. And you think, 'What did you work for?' I mean, did you work for—It's what you've been dealt. So you just have to deal with it. If I could find a little cheaper and a little better, I would do it, yes—because it'd last longer that way, the money would."*[486]

Once again, individuals and families may be less likely to discuss or adequately prepare for Morbidity Risk because it is a maudlin topic. It is far more fun to only think of retirement as the vacation reward for having worked for so many years. I held that mind-set in a prior book on financial planning: "Retirement should be a very long vacation, and sometimes clients need help to enjoy the fruits of their lives' labor."[487] Financial planners, accountants, investment advisors, insurance agents, and estate attorneys may all agree on having working families welcoming their thoughts of retirement as a vacation. Yet these professionals may then remind folks that even vacation planning involves considerations for length of stay, budget or costs, and the value of maintaining some flexibility for unknown weather or circumstances.

As a practitioner, the first time I publicly described a disconcerting wealth observation about the baby boomer generation was at a 2012 national retirement forum.[488] Invited to speak as a panelist, I sat alongside an envoy to the US Senate Finance Committee, and I explained how baby boomers often "feel wealthier" than they should because of their generation's movement from company pensions to 401k plans.

Figure 5

Composition of Total Individual Net Worth

Pre–Baby Boomer Generation   Baby Boomer Generation

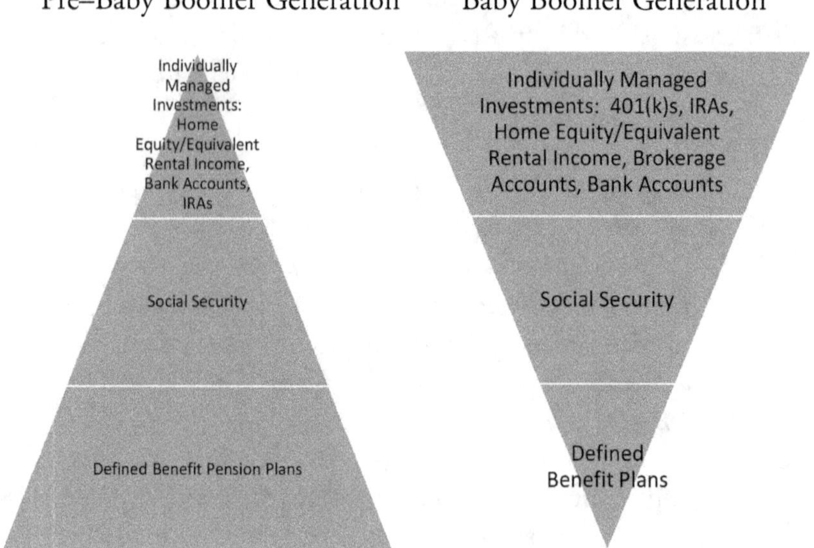

(Tiller, "Rock 'n' Roll to Rocking Chairs: Cognitively Impaired Baby Boomers' Impact and Liability for the Financial Industry," 2017)[489]

Now a practitioner-scholar, my previous concern remains—that baby boomers sometimes view statements for their IRA, 401k, 403b or other investments as "proof" (with pride and even amazement) of having amassed significantly higher net worth than their parents. Yet this perceived accomplishment is not true for many of them because they have not recognized the amount of wealth a lifetime pension represents. However, that calculation can easily be done in reverse—so pre-retirees can begin to realize how much they will need to accumulate to provide them with their own lifetime incomes.[490]

The term I originally coined to correct this suitability status oversight for both generations was—to calculate clients' "useable" net worth—later changed to a more apt description "effective net worth" or ENW. The aforementioned pre-retiree non-pensionaries, who are unaware of their ENW, may be inclined to save less, spend more, and end up less financially prepared for their future needs. Such individuals are not spendthrifts—they are merely unaware. Pension valuations are tracked closely by companies and regulators, but almost never by retirees or pre-retirees. Although divorce would be an exception—where pensions may be valued alongside the separating parties' investment statements.

Further ENW study may be warranted for scholarly economic discussion or practitioner calls to improve financial industry compliance and planning software.[491]

For future retirees, the important element is to understand their income assets, which will be relied upon in place of company pensions, could easily become compromised if needed for a long-term care illness such as Alzheimer's or dementia.

Figure 6

Preparation for these potential long-term care costs warrants discussions with family and qualified professionals on the following:

- **Asset allocation and prioritization**
- **Risk transference (i.e., LTC insurance)**
- **Alternative choices:**
  Government assistance (Medicaid and VA)
  Reverse mortgages (if not leaving home)
  Multigenerational homes

BEHIND THE CURTAIN

Creative Science

Researcher's Note

As a developing practitioner-scholar, I wanted my efforts to help bridge the gap between academia and practice. I decided to focus my final doctoral degree research project on Alzheimer's and the impending wave of cognitively impaired baby boomers. Even then, I knew my desire was to speak outside the academic audience who would be reviewing and evaluating my work. My respect for scholars was immense, but my years of study had shown me vast amounts of brilliant research in all fields is too often hidden away from the people who it might benefit the most. The gap exists because of rigor and language differences. Academics demand statements, contentions, or assertions to be rigorously researched and explained. However, their complex vocabulary and scientific jargon pose a language barrier for nonacademics to read their research. After three decades in the business world, I did not elect to go back to school to get a PhD (doctor of philosophy) in economics, finance, or behavioral studies. Aside from believing I was far too old to begin a university professorial tenure trek, I wanted to investigate and inform other professionals and the public on many of the business problems I had seen. For me, attaining a DBA (doctor of business administration) would develop my research skills while matching my intent to write to a broader audience.

My DBA program's choices for the final year's doctoral research deliverable included a traditional dissertation, but also a research-informed book. I chose the latter. The extra complexity for conceiving, conducting, and then converting a caregiver study into a credible, yet readable, text utilized much of what I had learned in both business and academics. Encouraged by my professors and fellow doctoral candidates, I found my research motivations enhanced each time others would tell me how Alzheimer's had touched their own lives. Their support earned my sincerest personal appreciation for being permitted to deliver this research to a public audience.

* * *

"Pay no attention to that man behind the curtain!"[492]

Nearly a century ago, those famous words—which bellowed through loudspeakers in the 1939 cinematic masterpiece *The Wizard of Oz*—showed a glimpse of a meager man trying to present a larger-than-life image of himself to the world. This classic film's example of an individual's intent to skew reality may explain much of our current society's challenge in recognizing what to believe. The items each of us see, read, or experience influence or shape our individual perceptions of the truth.

"Alternate facts," "fake news," and an endless onslaught of online and multimedia information make it difficult to recognize what is or is not valid. For a researcher, this communication challenge is dealt with by "pulling back the curtain"—for people to see the methodology behind the information. Allowing people to learn how their findings were derived—by the gathering, analyzing, and relating of data obtained through an unbiased scientific process. Academic researchers spend a great deal of their time focused upon these background details in their writings and discussions—yet the information presented to the public often excludes them from being welcomed "backstage."

Forgotten Faces: Family Caregiver Voices is an example of prescriptive research—intended to primarily inform the public. It was designed to explore the "caregiver to a cognitively impaired family member" problem facing millions of unsuspecting people. Then, to inform them on the findings—with a strict researcher's methodology, dutifully and ethically. Providing readers a behind-the-scenes vantage is part of a researcher's obligation, to disclose the process, as well as the data finding's strengths and weaknesses. When the reader is invited to see how the information was derived and reported—they should understand its trustworthiness.

The objective of this book is to create awareness, evoke empathy, and encourage action ahead of the anticipated wave of individuals becoming caregivers to a cognitively impaired family member as the baby boomers age. Therefore, the orientation of this research-informed book to inform a public audience ahead of other scholars altered its structure for relaying the data findings. Prioritizing communication to those who may someday be at, or near, the center of the caregiver to a cognitively impaired family member phenomenon was paramount. For this reason, the book design to report the research results was tailored into a somewhat inverted manner versus traditional academic writing:

Figure 7

Public Audience	Academic Audience
1) Acquaint reader with those who have already dealt with the problem	1) Define the problem scope and research gap warranting study
2) Explain why it is important for the reader to understand the problem	2) List the existing literature reviewed and prior researchers' findings
3) Show how the research was compiled and presented	3) State any theories or hypotheses and their foundational research
4) Reinforce important elements from the study	4) Summarize the method used and expected findings from the data
5) List citations and references with additional information	5) Display the data findings through case story presentation

Some of the scientific rigor behind the cases, challenges, and commentary displayed has purposefully been identified in the *Notes* section instead of within the text. To minimize disruption for the reader, small innocuous numbers are listed throughout the book's text. Each of these numbers corresponds to a *Notes* entry. Some entries are merely participant citations or references, while others are definitions, additional researcher commentary, or even examples of referenced documents. Providing these additional items which follow the text is to help prove to the reader the information conveyed was scientifically accurate.

Methods and Miles

While case study researchers customarily protect their subjects' identities, known as "masking," the family caregiver voices read throughout the text are genuine. All caregiver comments read were spoken by the research participants, not created by the researcher. The caregiver study conducted and methods used for reporting its results were more elaborate than apparent in the "Love Thy Stranger" case stories.

"Fred," "Janice," "Alice," and "Yvonne" were the representable faces given to embody the 24 actual caregivers' blended comments in the study. All participants' quotations read were specifically used in situational context, with changes only for masking purposes—not even allowing grammar or word choice alterations. The qualitative research[493] technique developed to allow their direct quotes to be layered and read as a continuing dialogue is the mosaic-exemplar poly vocal narrative method (MEPVN).[494] A brief diagram of the process appears below with a more detailed explanation in the *Notes* section.

Figure 8
Mosaic-Exemplar Poly Vocal Narrative (MEPVN) Method

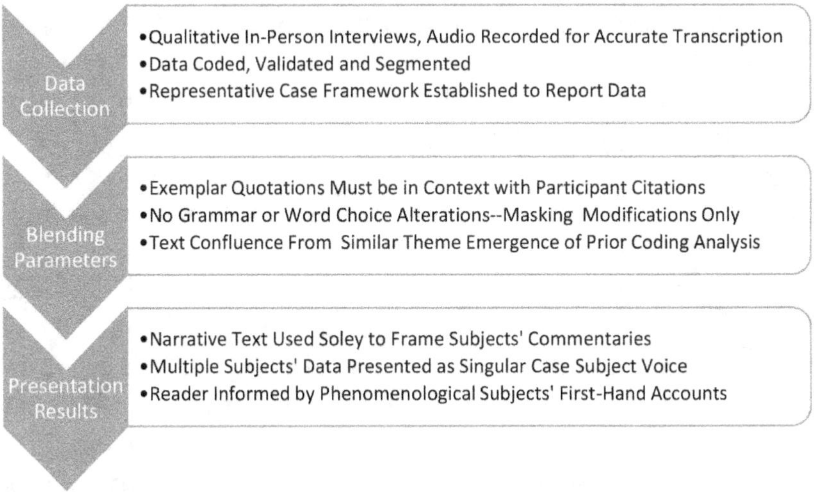

Sensitive case study research subjects' identities must be protected when relating the actual experiences of people. Therefore, participants' names, gender, or other identifying items are changed in order to keep them from being recognized.

The MEPVN process is simplistic in design, but was quite cumbersome to complete. Simply stated—it began with separating the interview audio transcript data into the different caregiver relationships with the cognitively impaired family members: husband caregiving for wife, wife caregiving for husband, child caregiving for parent, and a more distant relationship (reported as grandchild caring for grandparent).

Once segmented, the common or reoccurring themes that emerged from their families' stories were noted to determine which incidents, issues, or other items were experienced within each group. These included their comments about the prediagnosis behaviors, doctors' interactions, family discussions, wandering, care concerns, legal, financial, driving, incontinence, home care, facility, end-of-life decisions, etc.

A personalized identity embodying the caregiver characteristics for a majority of each study segment (i.e., "Fred," "Janice," "Alice," and "Yvonne") was chosen—with their circumstances, surroundings, and physical attributes representational to their respective group.

Even the pets' names, number, and/or species had to be altered to mask the participants' identities, but still matched the representative caregivers. Each personal story element shared by the four representative caregivers was an actual individual or blended quotation of one or more caregivers. These caregivers' own words were then carefully framed within a researcher narration to provide a continual conversational flow for the reader.

All interviews with the caregivers were conducted face-to-face. This allowed me to personally witness, then describe within the four case stories, an accurate representation of the 24 caregivers' actual pauses, inflections, emotional reactions—and even the pets' interactions—just as they had occurred during the study interviews.

Detailing these nonverbal cues was an important element to report with their comments. The interviews were emotionally charged regardless of gender or relationship segment—with very few subject participants not utilizing the tissues placed in front of them during each session.

Figure 9
Caregiver Case Segmentation and Research Writing Cycle

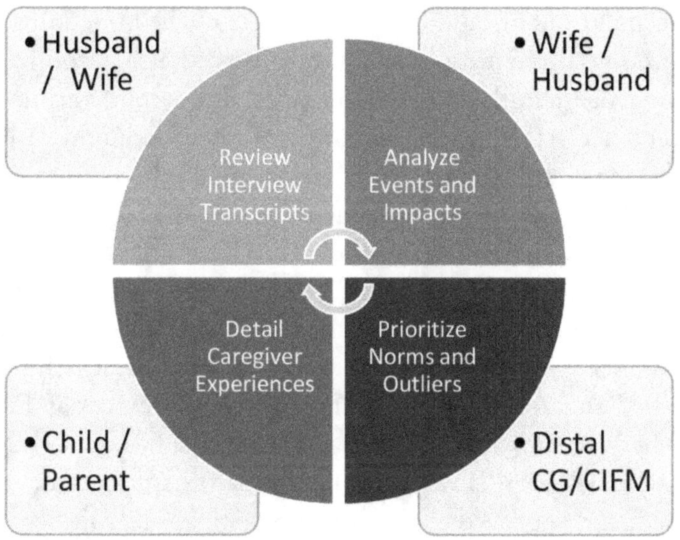

To confirm the information found in the interviews was an accurate reflection of what caregivers to a cognitively impaired family member may experience—I separately reviewed the transcripts of the four industry professionals who were interviewed independently. These industry professionals' identities were also required to be protected. Each of them has spent many years working directly with these types of caregivers—as support group facilitators or providing caregiver training.

Learning by firsthand account of another's actual experience increases one's ability to see the other person's perspective—especially if it differs from their own. Obtaining a proper perspective for understanding what is being communicated is vital to better perceive the accuracy, or truthfulness, of any assertion—for research or otherwise. Overt opinion, faulty data interpretation, and unintentional or intentional bias can undermine the credibility of research results.

While the data that will emerge from the research is unknown prior to its start—there first must be some focus upon what is to be studied and what may, or may not, be discovered.

Before anything else could be given consideration, a central research concern deserving attention was identified. As a practitioner-scholar intent on drawing awareness to the impending rise of cognitive impairment and family caregivers, the first consideration was *how* to best study the phenomenon. The second was to decide *what* audience(s) the information from the research should be directed toward. Finally, selecting *which* medium and method might best disclose that information to the targeted audience(s). These questions helped lead to the idea to study those who have already gone through the caregiver to a cognitively impaired family member experience in order to create awareness, evoke empathy, and advocate action.

To undertake the caregiver study, there was a research protocol established and approved to ensure appropriate respect and privacy would be given to the volunteer participant subjects. A university Institutional Review Board (IRB) proposal was discussed, drafted, amended, and approved ahead of any participant recruitment.

A demonstration that the research would be conducted with the study participants' well-being in mind was of great importance to the IRB. The existence of the IRB aids greatly in assuring the public that research is being conducted in accordance with the ethical standards developed over many decades.

Substantial rules exist to govern any "human research studies"[495] conducted. Their purpose is to help ensure individuals are voluntarily participating, made aware of the research purpose, and protected from harmful consequences that may benefit the researchers at the expense of the subjects.

This research study was identified as having "minimal risk" to the research volunteers, with no more harm than them speaking to friends or families about their experiences. The IRB was informed of my decades of tactfully discussing such matters with clients—and my expectation that the participants' interviews, although potentially emotional, would be somewhat cathartic for them. Yet to safeguard against a lingering heightened emotional issue for any participant—I informed the IRB that local professional support group contact information would be made available to each volunteer.

Within the IRB proposal was the Study Invitation/Flyer (Figure 10) to announce the research project and welcome contact from interested caregivers—both current and previous—to cognitively impaired family members.

Figure 10

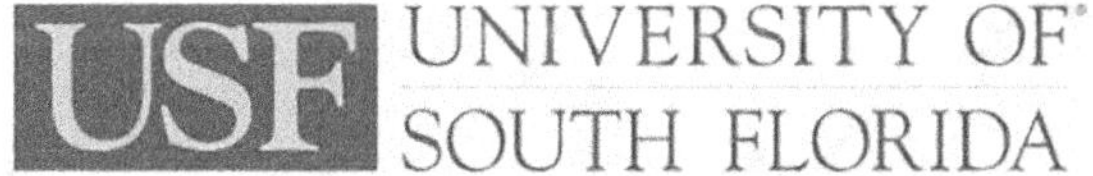

"Caregiver to a Cognitively Impaired Family Member Phenomenon"
IRB # 00030013

Current or previous caregivers to a family member with Alzheimer's, dementia or other cognitive impairment are respectfully welcomed to participate in a confidential research study to better inform future caregivers for similar roles.

Unfortunately, millions more Americans will also become caregivers to cognitively impaired family members. Your participation to share your own caregiver experiences may help this study's efforts to "create awareness," "evoke empathy" and "advocate action" to benefit those caregivers who will follow.

To participate in this research study, you would:

- **Volunteer to meet with a researcher for a 45-90 minute in-person confidential interview about your current or previous role as caregiver to a cognitively impaired relative.**
- **Be welcomed to have a family member or friend attend the interview with you.**
- **Receive contact information for a local caregiver support group for any further discussion(s) you may desire.**

To learn more or to become a part of this research study, please provide your contact information in confidence to the research team at: roberttiller@XXXX.XXX.XXX so additional study information may be sent. Thank you.

Also requiring approval before use were the study's "Consent Forms" for both the caregivers and the industry professionals.[496] The IRB proposal also included details on the purpose for gathering the data, the manner for collecting the data, protecting the data, and who else might have access to the confidential information of the study. Once satisfied that the study complied with the "Human Research Studies" requirements, the IRB gave approval (Figure 11) to move from preparation of the study to actually conducting it.

Figure 11

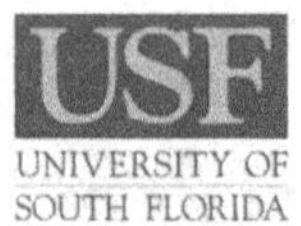

RESEARCH INTEGRITY AND COMPLIANCE
Institutional Review Boards, FWA No. 00001669
12901 Bruce B. Downs Blvd., MDC035 • Tampa, FL 33612-4799
(813) 974-5638 • FAX (813) 974-7091

April 7, 2017

Robert Tiller
COBA Executive Program
Tampa, FL 33612

RE: **Expedited Approval for Initial Review**
IRB#:   Pro00030013
Title: Caregiver to a Cognitively Impaired Family Member Phenomenon

Study Approval Period: 4/7/2017 to 4/7/2018

Dear Mr. Tiller:

On 4/7/2017, the Institutional Review Board (IRB) reviewed and **APPROVED** the above application and all documents contained within, including those outlined below.

Approved Item(s):
Protocol Document(s):

Study Protocol for Caregiver to a Cognitively Impaired Family Member Phenomenon Version#1-040417.docx

Consent/Assent Document(s)*:

CIFM Study#00030013 Industry Professionals Consent Form 040517.docx.pdf
CIFM Study#0030013 Caregiver Participant Consent Form 040517.docx.pdf

*Please use only the official IRB stamped informed consent/assent document(s) found under the "Attachments" tab. Please note, these consent/assent documents are valid until the consent document is amended and approved.

It was the determination of the IRB that your study qualified for expedited review which includes activities that (1) present no more than minimal risk to human subjects, and (2) involve only procedures listed in one or more of the categories outlined below. The IRB may review research through the expedited review procedure authorized by 45CFR46.110. The research proposed in this study is categorized under the following expedited review category:

(6) Collection of data from voice, video, digital, or image recordings made for research purposes.

(7) Research on individual or group characteristics or behavior (including, but not limited to, research on perception, cognition, motivation, identity, language, communication, cultural beliefs or practices, and social behavior) or research employing survey, interview, oral history, focus group, program evaluation, human factors evaluation, or quality assurance methodologies.

As the principal investigator of this study, it is your responsibility to conduct this study in accordance with IRB policies and procedures and as approved by the IRB. Any changes to the approved research must be submitted to the IRB for review and approval via an amendment. Additionally, all unanticipated problems must be reported to the USF IRB within five (5) calendar days.

We appreciate your dedication to the ethical conduct of human subject research at the University of South Florida and your continued commitment to human research protections. If you have any questions regarding this matter, please call 813-974-5638.

Sincerely,

John A. Schinka, Ph.D.

John Schinka, Ph.D., Chairperson
USF Institutional Review Board

Approval from the IRB allowed for participant recruitment to begin, then face-to-face caregiver interviews, in-person or telephone industry professional interviews, audio recordings to be transcribed, and data reviewed. What can now be so simply stated actually demanded months of preparation, hundreds of miles traveling, and hundreds more hours spent for the interviews: arranging, conducting, reading, and relistening and analyzing—followed by months of writing, editing, and rewriting. (See Figure 12)

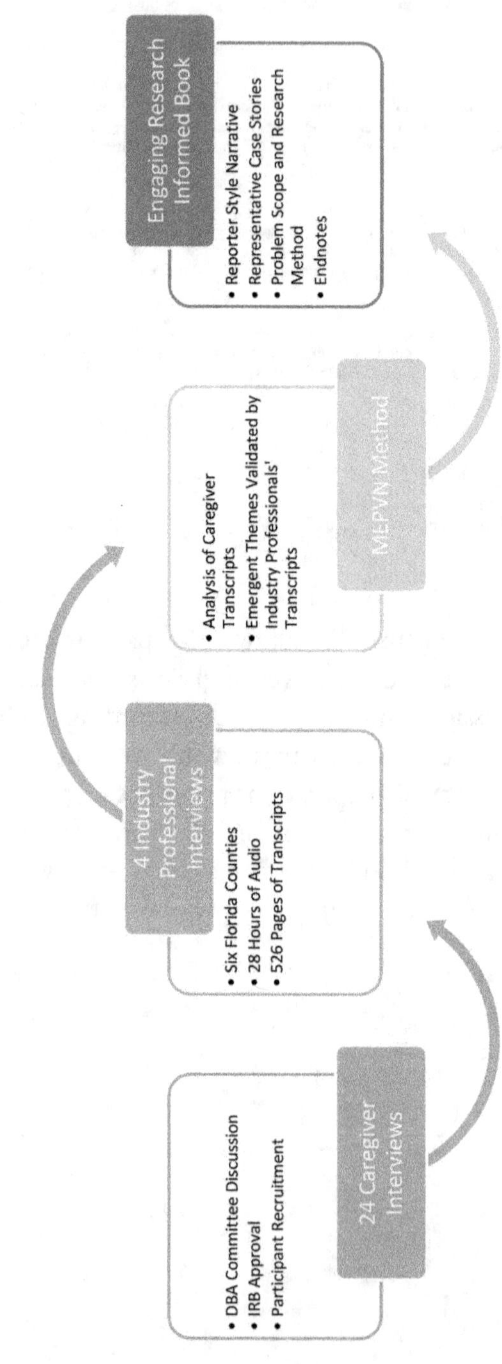

Figure 12
Research-Informed Dissertation Book Process
Engaging Research Informed Book
Reporter Style Narrative
Representative Case Stories
Problem Scope and Research Method
Endnotes
MEPVN Method
Analysis of Caregiver Transcripts
Emergent Themes Validated by Industry Professionals' Transcripts
4 Industry Professional Interviews
Six Florida Counties
28 Hours of Audio
526 Pages of Transcripts
24 Caregiver Interviews
DBA Committee Discussion
IRB Approval
Participant Recruitment

The identities of the caregiver and industry professional participants—along with the audio recordings, transcripts, data analysis, MEPVN methodology, book drafts, and *Notes* inclusions— were all made available to the dissertation research book project's cochairs.

These professors' access to the identifying information was disclosed on the participants' consent forms and necessary for them to attest to the validity of the research. They, along with the other people and organizations vital for completing this research project, are recognized in the *Acknowledgments*, ahead of the *Notes* section.

Limits and Outliers

The book's caregiver research study interviewed a very small sampling of the millions of caregivers in this country. While the accurate depiction of its results can help inform on the phenomenon, it does not represent every potential circumstance or feeling a caregiver may experience.

This limitation to the research is recognized so that the reader may elect to continue seeking a broader understanding than may be found within the scope of this study.

A few areas the study sample did not produce enough data to report on were the following:

- The impact of fewer financial resources on individuals' care and their families
- An ethnic comparative of differences or similarities
- The caregiver perspective of an Inappropriate Family Fiduciary

Researchers may be able to explore the first two areas more readily than the IFFs. Individuals with poor capabilities or bad intentions toward their ill family members are quite unlikely to volunteer to be interviewed about their caregiving. Should they admit committing elder abuse or financial exploitation to a researcher, it could exceed the level of confidentiality customarily granted to research subjects.

Another limit of this study was its intentional design to study the caregivers through only qualitative (text data) research and not to pursue quantitative (or statistical data) results. In part, this occurred by purposefully not using any previously established caregiver strain, burden, or coping survey questions.

To numbers-oriented researchers, the limited sample size (and different "caregiver stress" or "well-being" identifiers than the survey's language) makes a statistical comparison to any larger, less-intensive interview caregiver studies more challenging and less meaningful. However, unlike these much larger sample caregiver studies, the rationale for not using them was to give the caregiver participants broad latitude for expressing their personal experiences—in their own words with emotional detail.

I contend the case stories the study produced have accomplished that objective and would assert that such a face-to-face, deep-dive interview technique for a random sampling of future large telephone survey studies (even without this book's MEPVN method for reporting the data) is warranted to help affirm their results accurately capture the surveyed caregivers' true circumstances.

Data collected that appears to be outside of a studied sample's normal range of results are called *outliers* by researchers. While some of the outlier caregiver comments were not representative enough of this study's sample to become part of the case stories, they may still reflect the sentiment of other caregivers within the general population.

The study's industry experts' independent transcript comments affirmed the overall caregiver experience data that was collected and reported was within expected norms—or what should have been experienced by caregivers to a cognitively impaired family member.

One item mentioned by the industry experts which only appeared as an outlier in this study sample, only having a slight appearance within the caregivers' comments, was the challenge young children in caregiving households may bear:

> *"One of the kids at school one day said, 'Your*
> *dad looks kind of crazy,' because he showed up…*
> *and his hair was all sticking out because he hadn't*

really groomed himself that day. And I never talked about it, because I never thought anybody could really identify with it."[497]

* * *

"There was one time where we came home and he had pooped and had not realized it, and had sat in various chairs in the house, and it was just everywhere. He was covered in it, furniture was covered in it, and that was, for me, the moment where it was like, 'I need Mom to come home and do this, because I am not comfortable putting my dad in the shower and washing him.' I could clean the sofa; I just was not comfortable caring for him in that way. So she came home and took care of him and actually insisted on cleaning everything. She wouldn't let us touch anything."[498]

A few of the study's caregivers were quite candid on a subject that was also not representational enough to be included in the case stories: "euthanasia" or "the right to die." As an unbiased researcher, I cannot simply omit reporting a less significant finding within the data because it may be disturbing or did not fit within the representational case studies—hence their inclusion here:

"I would have wanted to probably call Dr. Kevorkian. Really. I would not have wanted to live in that fashion. You asked me what I wanted. That would have been my decision."[499]

* * *

"I would want them to let me kill myself. I really—I think that...I really, really believe this, that when you reach a point with Alzheimer's or any other disease, where you no longer have a quality of

life, I think it would be much kinder if you let that person go with assisted suicide, so they don't have to die alone… The last thing in the world I want is my sister to have to take care of me. She's got a life, a good life, she doesn't need that. If I don't have a life anymore, what's the point? I'm just taking air in. I feel like that very, very strongly and I don't understand why we can't do that."[500]

* * *

"They put down horses and animals and things, but elderly people that there's no life to it all—'No, we can't do that. You have to tough it out.' And I think that's totally wrong. But that's only my opinion."[501]

* * *

"I can understand why, especially these older couples, why they murder-suicide. I can totally understand it, totally, because you are so backed into a corner emotionally, financially—You can't see a window to crawl out of, and you don't want to be without your spouse either. I can understand that. I can totally. It's not something that I thought of, but I can understand it, especially the people in their 80s and 90s—I completely can understand it, and I don't blame them. I don't blame them."[502]

* * *

"I would have him sell my house, move to Oregon, and let me take a handful of pills—to save both of us."[503]

* * *

"Visit some of these dementia wards and look at some of these people. Why not give the right to die thing if that's what they want? If they don't want it, that's fine. It's a voluntary thing, but some of the condition these people are in, it's shameful the way that they have to go on…It may sound harsh or something, but that's my opinion."[504]

Other outliers simply addressed items that were somewhat contrary to, or outside the focus of, the majority of the caregiver study participants' comments:

"I think they need to be educated in the doctor's office how to help coach that caregiver in order to get the care to the individual—so the caregiver is not breaking down, or not having difficulties just to get things going."[505]

* * *

"If she sees somebody else having joy, that makes her happy. She doesn't understand why she's happy, but I truly believe it's because that is how she's just always been. I love to see her smile."[506]

* * *

"She said that if God meant animals to live in houses, they would have hands like carpenters so they could build them."[507]

Researcher's Note

I hope the unique structure of Forgotten Faces: Family Caregiver Voices *helps to build awareness for a broader audience than might otherwise have investigated this research area. In its development, there were two pivotal creative art items that helped decide its purpose and form.*

The first was when I hoped to persuade my professors to endorse my nontraditional doctoral dissertation deliverable choice by adding music and videos to my formalized research proposal. Mine featured a song by Cameron Washburn[508]—a gifted songwriter and my brother-in-law, whose lyrics artistically chronicle the world around him. Behind his soulful vocal is a beautiful love song, masked as a rock ballad called Time to Share. *It tells how a couple's bond, forged over a lifetime, is still too strong to be erased by Alzheimer's. Throughout the compilation of this book, I would listen to its soothing tone and powerful message.*

The second item was a brief but inspiring encounter with a neuroscientist that cemented my decision to have the caregivers themselves inform the reader. Preparing to attend the 2017 Alzheimer's Association's International Conference in London, I read Dr. Lisa Genova would be speaking at one of the evening events. Dr. Genova is recognized as the best-selling author of the novel and movie Still Alice—*a fictional depiction of a Harvard professor's experience in dealing with early onset Alzheimer's disease. It is a bit unsettling, quite touching, and very informative. I had the opportunity to hear Dr. Genova talk about her motivation for writing* Still Alice *and was fortunate enough to briefly speak with her afterward. I was inspired by how she combined her scientific knowledge and her personal family connection to Alzheimer's into the motivation that helped her to produce a captivating and thought-provoking story.*

While I cannot craft such a musical tribute or envision a fictionalized account that would match these caregivers' actual experiences—I do hope this book engages, informs, and encourages those individuals and families who will travel their own Alzheimer's journeys to share their time well.

RESEARCH REFLECTIONS

Lessons and Opportunities

Researcher's Note

In many ways, I found it a great challenge to separate my feelings from the study participant caregivers' experiences during our meetings. It was imperative that I followed my strict study protocol and methodology to avoid researcher bias from tainting their data and lowering the scientific credibility of the results. What each of the volunteer participants was unaware of before or during our interviews was that I shared many of their personal reasons for wanting to see this topic explored in front of a broad public audience.

My wife and I spent several years at the epicenter of the family caregiver pond. We became direct stakeholders in the phenomenon ourselves when my father-in-law had dementia while my mother-in-law had Alzheimer's.

Like the study's family caregivers, we too dismissed early warning signs, struggled with phone calls, role reversal, taking away car keys, increased health challenges, home care aides, assisted living moves, visitations, doctors, hospitals, medical billings, hospice, funerals, guilt, frustration, grieving, and estate issues. I learned you may not see the stakeholder ripples on the pond from the center because while you are there, you are focused upon just staying afloat—grabbing onto the nearest item demanding attention, then another, and another, and another.

If I grew up between my Mamaw's, grandfather's, and clients' Alzheimer's journeys, I grew old with my in-laws' experience. The fitting axiom then became "older and wiser." For when the ripples ceased, and the pond was still—reflection and healing followed.

This book was published to help educate and encourage current and future direct stakeholders who are, or may be, at the center of the Alzheimer's pond—as caregiver or the family member needing care. My hope is that it will also enlighten less direct and indirect stakeholders—family members, friends, neighbors, coworkers, doctors, industry leaders, researchers, and policymakers throughout our expansive society.

* * *

A prescriptive research effort is intended to properly study and disclose its findings on a problem deemed worthy of attention. A successful prescriptive research effort will either find solutions, identify action areas, or detect what deserves further research.

"Love Thy Stranger" provided actual family caregivers' words for a better understanding of their experiences.

"Rock 'n' Roll to Rocking Chairs" called attention to the wave of baby boomers who will become cognitively impaired and areas to be considered by future caregivers and those around them.

"Behind the Curtain" described the trustworthy nature of the data presented, the limitations of the case study, and the disciplined scientific path followed in this book's compilation.

"Research Reflections" recaps the most important issues—with both researcher and caregiver commentary.

Forgotten Faces: Family Caregiver Voices has allowed caregivers themselves to be the primary source of informing readers—so it closes with their advice to future caregivers, to other stakeholders, and to their own caregivers (if cognitively impaired themselves).

This research began with a conceptual scheme[509] that caregivers to a cognitively impaired family member may be unprepared and overwhelmed. The data provided from this caregiver study affirms that may be true for most, but also offers hope that with education, adequate support, and embracing positive coping skills—people can be better prepared and less overwhelmed.

The facts are clear, the challenges have been noted—but finding solutions for the public, policymakers, and other researchers are beyond the scope of this book. Therefore, readers are encouraged to remember the lessons found in this research, while they take action—addressing the concerns that may most affect them.

Accepting the possibility of an unpleasant circumstance, followed by action to avert it or minimize its severity, can be applied by each of the book's three intended audiences—the public, policymakers, and researchers. Ahead of the upcoming wave of baby boomer cognitive impairment, each audience has an opportunity to ponder the following questions, then continue or improve their efforts:

Public

Where and what care would they or their family members need, desire, or be able to afford in the event of a cognitive impairment?

How can they better prepare themselves for the possibility of an impairment predicament—legally, financially, and emotionally?

Where should they look for establishing an adequate caregiver support network, and who should be named to handle the medical, financial, and legal affairs as primary, contingent, or tertiary fiduciaries?

Policymakers

How can the present Medicare/Medicaid system accommodate all those afflicted and affected?

What changes or reforms are appropriate to support individuals and families for long-term care?

How can efforts to constrain Elder Financial Exploitation be accomplished without creating an undue further burden for earnest caregivers?

Researchers

What causes these ailments—and which medications, behavioral changes, or other treatments could eradicate their existence or improve living with them before then?

What will be the full financial impact for individuals, industry, and state or federal governments, and what solutions are available?

How can *both* care for the cognitively impaired and support systems for their caregivers be improved—at the medical, financial, and social sciences levels?

Caregivers' Advice

To Future Caregivers

"The whole 'do things in advance' is a big thing…get good advice and to put as many of these things into place, the documents and so forth…as early as possible. In addition, I would say, set your priorities very carefully, figure out what's the important part, and forgive yourself for all of the other things."[510]

* * *

"Be prepared, have a lot of patience, be very tolerant and accepting, accepting their wide variables that they have that comes with them."[511]

* * *

"I think financial condition is very important, especially, and I've seen money cause a lot of fight and tensions in the household. Then I would still say, just be in touch with friends—you need a circle too, because there will be a lot of naysayers and 'putting you down people'—but you need somebody to uplift you, somebody to encourage you and you need to have that support system so that you can talk to people."[512]

* * *

"It's a disease. It's not something to be ashamed of."[513]

* * *

"Every journey is different, but to be aware that the one you know, and that you love, is going to continue to change, and some days the person will be wonderful, and other times, they may be more confused, and the best thing to do is not argue with them. Agree with them or divert them."[514]

* * *

"Dignity—that they still deserve to have as much dignity as they can. My mom, even though she doesn't remember who she is, I still remember and I still have to respect and love and honor all of that. If you have to find someplace else to put them, it needs to be some place where she'll be treated with dignity."[515]

To Family and Friends

"You don't want to force someone to step away and say, 'Okay, you can't go down there. You can't do this. You can't do that.' Then down the road they're going to feel guilty because they didn't do what they really felt that they should do."[516]

* * *

"I think you want to try and have the conversations with the family as to maybe what they can do to help, 'If *you* take a trip down for me—I would feel comfortable not going.'…I think a lot of times people don't talk about it, that's the problem. When they don't realize *why* you're doing what you're doing, and maybe…there's some things someone else could do to help.

There's got to be more conversation—I think it's the problem."[517]

* * *

"I think the friends should reach out, not… asking, 'Do you need help for caregiving?' The friends should reach out, maybe cook a meal, take the kids out, come and say, 'Hey, why don't you go take a shower?'"[518]

* * *

"As a friend of someone, I wouldn't wait until they ask for help…don't even question. They do need help in some way. Even doing grocery shopping, or bringing a meal over, or offering to stay with a loved one for an hour or two is tremendously helpful."[519]

* * *

"One thing that impressed me this year, we had six new people show up (to support group meeting) at the same time one day. They were neighbors of a couple where she was starting to have signs, and they were coming to find out how do they deal with it…And that's what people need I think…then…be it a parent and a child, or a couple will have help to get through this thing. They aren't out there by themselves."[520]

* * *

"Help them in any way…Just be there for them…Cook a meal, help with the cleaning or have somebody do some simple chores—because those simple chores are not simple when you are taking care of somebody."[521]

To Employers

"I think the needs of a caregiver in this situation are equal to that of a newborn or perhaps more, because you never know what the day's going to bring with the situation. They might be having a great day and getting yourself off to work is not a problem or they might be having a terrible day and you can't leave them."[522]

* * *

"Being a small business person, I see both sides…I see that someone not being at my place of business has a huge effect on my business because I'm a small business, but I can also see it from the side that there are days that my mom just can't be left alone."[523]

* * *

"Give them the same consideration for that person as if it was a child that they had. If I need to take off time to take my mother to the doctor, I need you to be as okay with that as if I would say, 'Okay. It's time for the baby's six-month checkup or whatever.' People don't understand that. 'Well, don't you have somebody else to take them?' 'No, I don't. I really don't. It's me.'"[524]

* * *

"Believe me, they'd rather be at work any day of the week—then to have to deal with that. I don't know what an employer would do…In order for me to stay, if there was—a daycare in their office like for children."[525]

* * *

"I think these companies…with billions of dollars of cash in the banks, that they're not reinvesting into society. They certainly could be doing a whole lot more."[526]

* * *

"People in my generation are the 'sandwich generation.' Even younger than me, but they still work, and they've got kids, and they've got the parents, and you can't do it all. You can't do it all. It's too much. I don't know. I don't know what I'd tell employers. I don't know. It's a tough job. Tough job."[527]

To Policymakers

"Expand in-home health coverage…To think that all the baby boomers—10,000 a day turning 65—who are going to come down with some related dementia or other disease are going to be able to go to a nursing home is ridiculous. It's going to be an epidemic."[528]

* * *

"The people in government don't understand the necessity of having respite care for the caregivers that are taking care of these peo-ple. They get worn out. They get burnout. This needs to be something that's covered for them. Get them three hours a week to just get out of the house. Let the daughter go get her hair done. Let the son go play golf, go bowling, whatever it is. They need to know that they've got some-body there watching their loved one and that they're able to just think about themselves for a second."[529]

* * *

"Non-medical home care…not just with the cognitive impairment but with any senior… One hour…once a month to put a bowl on a top shelf, prevent them from getting onto a stepstool and falling off and breaking a hip. That's preven-tative care. How much money have I just saved the government because now they don't have to pay for the hip replacement, the hospital stay, the surgery, the rehab afterwards? If they would learn to just pay for one hour."[530]

* * *

"They need quality care for their loved one, which you cannot always do at home. I mean, if they become bedridden, if they become inconti-nent, physically you can't do all of that, so you need assistance either at home or in a nursing home, and no one family has enough money to do that, and they need help. They need help."[531]

* * *

"I know when I was younger, I lived in an ideal world and you respected politicians…Now, our country is so divided. Just, 'I'm right—you're wrong,' 'No, I'm right—you're wrong,' and they don't work together…I've tried sending emails to politicians…My first series of letters was to work together, compromise…don't just vote the party line because you're Republican or a Democrat. Most of them didn't even respond."[532]

To Their Own Caregivers (If Cognitively Impaired Themselves)

"I don't want them to be overwhelmed, so my concern is more on them. I know I'll be taken care of. I know that between the five kids we've got, at least one of them will take care of us. But I don't want to be a burden on them, so we're trying to make sure everything is set that we're not."[533]

* * *

"The younger daughter said, 'Shady Pines.' I know I saw that on *Golden Girls* somewhere… Yeah, Shady Pines, that's what they always threaten me with. 'Shady Pines, Mom!' Other than that, I don't think we've had an honest discussion with them—but maybe that's something we need to think about."[534]

* * *

"I want them to know, and I've told them, 'Find me a good, comfortable home. Don't stress yourself over me. Don't try and do what I did, because I'm not going to know the difference.'

And, what's important—(crying)—is that they take care of themselves. I said, 'Come visit. Make sure I'm not being mistreated, but make sure I'm being taken care of—but don't try and do that. Don't do what I did.'"[535]

* * *

"Geez, just be kind. Be kind. There were times when I should have been kinder…because my expectations were too high."[536]

* * *

"I would hope that they would still treat me like me. I love to sing, and I love to go to concerts where people sing, and I would hope that somebody could take me to concerts, and not just keep me in the house, even though I may not have a clue what's happening—but there could be that little tiny glimmer where I know."[537]

* * *

"Treat me with dignity, love and respect. I think the biggest thing that I learned with caregiving…was about keeping the atmosphere peaceful…The ability to know that you're being cared for—a hug…music, here's some tea, kindness gestures, and the emotional connection never got lost. It stayed there. I would want someone to connect with me like that."[538]

ACKNOWLEDGMENTS

This book was possible because of the heartfelt sharing of the family caregiver study participants—whose hope was their stories might enlighten caregivers and those around them, while encouraging doctors, researchers, politicians, and industry leaders to keep them in mind. My thanks to the Alzheimer's Family Organization, the USF Byrd Alzheimer's Institute, and the Alzheimer's Association for their assistance in recruiting volunteers, their databases, and their ongoing missions.

I thank my wife, Linda, for her ongoing support of my scholarly endeavors; and my parents, Bill and Ann, for their lifelong example and unwavering belief in me. My sisters, my friends, and my business associates—Irene, Jeanene, Dottie and Mel are thanked for their accommodating actions with my schedule.

My respect and appreciation are extended to the University of South Florida MUMA College of Business DBA program's creators and faculty who broadened my knowledge base and research abilities to provide me a greater voice as a practitioner-scholar. A noted "thank you" goes out to MUMA's dean, Dr. Moez Limayem, for giving the DBA program life; to Dr. Matthew Mullarkey, for his practitioner-scholar guidance and direction; and special thanks to program visionary Dr. T. Grandon Gill, whose passion for enhancing the informing sciences will affect generations to come. Also to my dissertation committee advisors: Dr. Moez Limayem, Dr. Paul Spector, Dr. Richard Plank, and especially my cochairs: Dr. Anand Kumar and Dr. Richard Will, as well as the entire MUMA staff, especially Michele and Lauren.

The final acknowledgment is for my fellow inaugural USF MUMA DBA cohort members:

Dr. Privin Alexander	Dr. Scott Hopes	Dr. Dana Parks
Dr. Charles Arant	Dr. Elizabeth Kerns	Adj. Prof. Lauren Rudd
Dr. Janene Culumber	Dr. Troy Montgomery	Dr. Natayla Sabga
Dr. Allen Deserranno	Dr. Timothy Novak	Dr. Rebecca Smith
Dr. Gilbert Gonzales	Dr. Christopher Olson	Brig. Gen. David Snyder
Dr. Robert Hammond	Dr. Steven Oscher	Dr. James Stikeleather
Dr. Mohamad Ali Hasbini	Dr. Timothy Papp	Dr. John Townsend

Their collective intelligence and multi-industry perspectives were paramount in my DBA journey. I am honored to know them and welcome their future achievements.

NOTES

Foreword

[1] 2017 CIFM Study, Institutional Review Board # 0030013, University of South Florida, Primary Investigator: Robert Tiller, DBA ('17) Candidate, MUMA College of Business.

[2] *Forgotten Faces: Family Caregiver Voices* developed the Mosaic-Exemplar Poly Vocal Narrative Method (MEPVN) to use the Qualitative Research Reporter Style for accurately and empathetically presenting data from 24 individual caregivers and 4 industry professional interview participants within four segmented case stories. The book explores the phenomenon of caregiving to a cognitively impaired family member from different subject perspectives: husband for wife, wife for husband, child for parent, and a more distal relationship. Similar to a written documentary, the text is framed as a research interview, dialogue-driven, first-person account of the investigation itself. This method and style provides an intensive level of subjects' thoughts and emotions to candidly inform the reader on the phenomenon.

Mosaic-Exemplar Poly Vocal Narrative Method / Qualitative Research Reporter Style:

 Construct: Blended multiple subject data, formatted into a representative case story as a single voice, through extensive, nearly exclusive use, of participants' exemplar quotations.

     Narrative text used solely to frame and bond the subjects' commentary so phenomenological informing is presented firsthand by the case participants themselves.

 Parameters: Subject quotations presented must accurately reflect the participant's context.

     Removal of extraneous words within quotes must be demonstrated through use of ellipses.

     Each full or partial quotation must be cited by participant number within text, footnotes or *Notes*.

> Full or partial clauses, including desirable phraseology of fragmented quotations, cannot be presented within case text espousing a differing subject perspective to that of the quoted party.
>
> Masking modifications for gender, names, tense, locale, or other participant identifiers aside, subject quotations must be genuine—without grammar and word choice corrections or alterations.
>
> Content suitable for text confluence must have emerged from similar themes identified during the qualitative research data coding process.

3   An inverted case design was selected to enhance readability and progression through the information being presented. (See "Behind the Curtain.")

4   Multiple audience objectives and considerations (from doctoral proposal).

5   A practitioner scholar is a "new breed of researcher coming into focus," doctorates, whose "research is driven by real business problems that can benefit from research, not by gaps or inconsistencies in the academic literature," Professor T. Grandon Gill, director of the MUMA DBA program, University of South Florida (K Morelli, *MUMA College of Business*, Nov. 15, 2016).

6   At the completion of a doctorate program, the candidates prepare a final deliverable that will demonstrate their acquired skills from their years of study—most often a dissertation or thesis. These are generally lengthy, complex research papers on a well-focused study topic. The Doctorate of Business Administration degree program at the MUMA College of Business is intent on educating practitioner-scholars, encouraging doctoral candidates to incorporate their research skills into final deliverables that might also draw from their years of executive business experience. Dissertations, a series of journal articles, a research-informed book, and a body of collective works could all be proposed by the DBA doctoral candidates. Upon approval of my cochairs and dissertation committee, this book was my chosen final dissertation project. The project's design and development, and the caregiver research study conducted, were monitored and reviewed by them throughout the progress.

7   See "About the Author."

8   Prescriptive research stems from research design action modeling whereby exploratory research is intended to impact future direction or products. However, this book has prioritized a public audience over academia; therefore, it seeks to explore and inform to impact readers', policymakers', and other researchers' actions.

Love Thy Stranger

9   Qualitative research involves the analysis of text data (such as interview transcripts and observational notes on subjects by the investigator) to under-

stand a phenomenon. It is "heavily dependent" upon the researcher's personal subject knowledge, analytic skills, and creative investigatory ability to apply an "ethically enlightened and participant-in-context attitude" to a strategic method of analysis. (Bhattacherjee, A., *Social Science Research: Principles, Methods, and Practices*, 2012)

10   See *Note* 495, Figures 17–19.

11   Brain scan (image pending)

12   A phenomenon is a common behavior, event, condition, or other problem for multiple people whose combined description of the experience may create a better understanding of it. (Creswell, J., *Qualitative Inquiry & Research Design*, 2007)

13   For data collection and reporting to be considered scientific research, it must both contribute to "a body of science" and "follow the scientific method." This book is an example of social science as it is a study of people experiencing a phenomenon. The scientific design and methods followed are discussed in "Behind the Curtain." (Bhattacherjee, A., *Social Science Research: Principles, Methods, and Practices*, 2012)

14   See "About the Author."

15   *Forgotten Faces: Family Caregiver Voices*

16   Participant CG 0027

17   Ibid.

18   Participant CG 0024

19   "Concentrated listening" and "engaged interest in what is being said" are important interviewer traits when pursuing effective questioning. (Seidman, Irving, *Interviewing as Qualitative Research*, 4th ed., 2013, page 95)

20   Participant CG 0010

21   Participant CG 0023

22   Participant CG 0016

23   Participant CG 0023

24   To ensure the data being collected through the caregiver study interviews was being accurately interpreted—I also interviewed four industry professionals with many years of direct experience dealing with caregivers to Alzheimer's and dementia situations. The interviews with these caregiver support group leaders/facilitators and/or caregiving trainers were separately analyzed to identify keywords and issues caregivers generally experience. The results validated the data from the caregiver study participants, while showing areas the study sample did not include. These limitations to the study are explained in "Behind the Curtain."

25   Participant IP 0032

26   See "Behind the Curtain."

27   Participant CG 0017

28   Ibid.

29   Participant CG 0019

30   Participant CG 0014

31   Participant CG 0003

32   *Covering* is a term used to describe the common ability for individuals with Alzheimer's or dementia to behave so others may not recognize they have a cognitive ailment. Prior to diagnosis, this behavior may delay recognition of their ailment. Several study participants described both early and midstage Alzheimer's-afflicted individuals covering too. Some had enough conversational abilities that people did not always realize they did not fully understand what they were speaking about—or, in some cases, to whom they were speaking. While others, already residing in lockdown wards or memory care units, were able to mask their ailments sufficiently to fool visitors and exit through an open door.

33   Participant CG 0003

34   Participant CG 0014

35   Participant CG 0011

36   Participant CG 0026

37   *Masking* is the process used to protect case study participants' identities. Case study subjects' identities are customarily held in confidence by the researcher. Beyond keeping access to identifiable data (e.g., contact lists, consent forms, interview transcripts) from anyone other than those disclosed on the consent forms, the data within the transcripts itself is put through a masking process. This entails "substituting" pseudonyms for people, places, or things that, left unchanged, could compromise a case study subject's identity. (Seidman, Irving, *Interviewing as Qualitative Research,* 4th ed., 2013, page 70)

38   See "Behind the Curtain."

39   See "Behind the Curtain."

40   Participants CG 0021/0022

41   Participant 0002

42   Participants CG 0021/0022

43   Participant CG 0013

44   Ibid.

45   Participant CG 0004

46   Participants CG 0021/0022

47   Participant CG 0006

48   Ibid.

49   *Senior moments* are often laughed at as momentary memory lapses attributed to getting older (e.g., forgetting what one walked into a room to get, not being able to recall a name midsentence, etc.). These moments are quite common and do not necessarily indicate an approaching Alzheimer's or dementia cognitive impairment, nor even mild cognitive impairment. However, a collective of odd memory lapses recognized by others may warrant a discus-

sion with a doctor. (Source: Beckwith, B., *Managing Your Memory: Practical Solutions for Forgetting*, 2004/2010)

50. Participant CG 0009

51. Ingersoll-Dayton, Starrels, and Dowler, "Caregiving for Parent and Parents-in-Law: Is Gender Important?" *The Gerontologist*, Vol. 36, No. 4, 483–491, 1996.

52. Participants CG 0021/0022

53. Ibid.

54. Participant CG 0006

55. Participant CG 0026

56. See "Storm Warning."

57. Participant CG 0006

58. Participants CG 0021/0022

59. Ibid.

60. Ibid.

61. Participant CG 0008

62. Participant CG 0033

63. Ibid.

64. Ibid.

65. Ibid.

66. Participant CG 0030

67. Participant CG 0007

68. Ibid.

69. Participant CG 0033

70. Participant CG 0008

71. Participant CG 0033

72. Participant CG 0024

73. Ibid.

74. Participant CG 0023

75. *Mini-Mental State Examination (MMSE),* also known as the *Folstein* test, is a short (10 question, 30-point) exam doctors use to measure a patient's cognitive abilities. Questions help to assess the patient's "orientation" (knowledge of their town, county or the season), "registration" (ability to recognize and repeat three unrelated words stated by the physician), "attention and calculation" (counting backward by sevens), "recall" (ability to restate the previous three words), and "language and Praxis" (recognizing time from a wristwatch and following instructions for: folding paper, writing, copying a drawing, etc.). (Source: http://www.fammed.usouthal.edu/Guides&JobAids/Geriatric/MMSE.pdf from Folstein, Folstein & McHugh, 1975, "Mini-mental state: A practical method for grading the cognitive state of patients for the clinician," *Journal of Psychiatric Research*, 1975; 12:189-198.)

76. Participant CG 0027

77. Participant CG 0015

78   Participant CG 0023
79   Participant CG 0026
80   Participant CG 0017
81   Ibid.
82   Ibid.
83   Participant CG 0019
84   Participant CG 0014
85   Participant CG 0002
86   Participant CG 0013
87   Participant CG 0002
88   Participant CG 0004
89   Participant CG 0006
90   Participant CG 0004
91   Participant CG 0023
92   Participant CG 0009
93   Participant CG 0013
94   Licensed practical nurse (LPN). Many assisted living facilities and nursing homes use LPNs to help care for the residents' required medical care beyond the non-nursing skill level convalescent custodial care, which may be performed by nurses' aides. Registered nurses (RNs) may handle more advanced care than LPNs and have completed a multiple-year educational, degreed program beyond the educational regimen for the often non-degreed certification of an LPN.
95   Participant CG 0008
96   Ibid.
97   Caregiver strain may bring on issues to be discussed with a medical doctor. Prescriptions are among the treatment options regularly needed to alleviate the symptoms. One of the study's industry professionals commented: "There's a variety of reactions depending on the individual, but some become stressed and anxious, depressed, frustrated…those are the biggies." Participant IP 0032
98   Ibid.
99   Ibid.
100   Participant CG 0033
101   Participant CG 0008
102   Ibid.
103   Participant CG 0033
104   Ibid.
105   Ibid.
106   Ibid.
107   Participant CG 0027
108   Participant CG 0023
109   Participant CG 0016

110   Industry Professional on support group purpose for caregivers:

> "They may be having problems with certain behaviors and people who have gone through that give them some suggestions. They get validated for their feelings, their frustrations, their emotions. Sometimes you could be angry and you feel guilty for being angry. They're dealing with a lot of guilt and it gives them support to go through that. You're watching this intelligent individual lose all their cognitive ability—it's very overwhelming.
>
> Going to a support group gives them someone who understands what they're going through. They get a hug, they get someone who says, 'I understand and I know how hard it is and I commend you,' and getting suggestions. They get suggestions for home care to go to, suggestions for doctors, telling them things, 'Oh, you need to get this in place. I didn't do it, you need to do this.' I think getting advice from that group is advice well taken because these are people that are doing it. It's not just someone telling them, who's a family member, it's somebody who walked the same path." (Participant IP 0001)

111   Participant CG 0027

112   Participant CG 0024

113   Ibid.

114   Ibid.

115   Participant CG 0023

116   Participant CG 0010

117   Respite may be home care aides, adult day care, support groups with separate supervised rooms for the ill, family, friends—any type of outside help that gives the caregiver a temporary break from their responsibilities. "Despite the high need for support, only 10 to 15 percent of caregivers use respite services, adult day services and support." (Alzheimer's Association, *Research Grants* 2006, www.alz.org, September 2017)

118   "Hospice care is a specialized kind of holistic care that comforts people of all ages and diagnoses when a cure is no longer possible. It is provided in many settings by interdisciplinary teams of expert professionals and trained volunteers who ease the physical, emotional and spiritual pain and stress of patients and families. It is most beneficial during the last six months of life. While palliative care focuses on additional medical support and comfort alongside curative care for many years of any illness." (Suncoast Hospice website: suncoasthospice.org, September 2017)

119   Participant CG 0024

120   Ibid.

121   Ibid.

122   Ibid.

123   Participant CG 0027

124   Ibid.

125   Ibid.

126   I was introduced by a caregiver support group facilitator to the members before their meeting's discussion began. Prior to the meeting, the leader thought it might help my research if I sat in to listen to their discussion. I thanked her for the welcome, but explained that doing so might make any members not interested in participating in the research study uncomfortable. Therefore, I had purposefully eliminated "observational" support group data collection from my study's recruitment design and formal research proposal. Instead, I distributed the approved study invitation/flyer, briefly told them I would be conducting individual, confidential interviews with family caregivers, and welcomed them to volunteer. Then, I thanked the group facilitator, the attendees, and left before any personal discussions began. Several individuals from the group did volunteer for the study—with none made aware of the others participating.

127   Participant CG 0003

128   Ibid.

129   Participant CG 0026

130   Participant CG 0003

131   Participant CG 0014

132   Participant CG 0017

133   Participant CG 0003

134   Ibid.

135   Ibid.

136   Participant CG 0026

137   Participant IP 0032

138   Participant CG 0011

139   Participant CG 0026

140   Participant CG 0011

141   "Alzheimer's Family Organization (AFO) is a community based, non-profit 501 (c) 3 organization focused on helping caregivers achieve and maintain a better quality of life not only for their loved ones, but for themselves." They serve eight Florida counties, offering caregiver learning and professional education for those working with Alzheimer's- and dementia-afflicted individuals, emergency placement assistance, respite care, and caregiver support groups. Their motto: "Family is our Middle Name." (Alzheimer's Family Organization website: alzheimersfamily.org, September 2017)

142   Participant CG 0014

143   Ibid.

144   Participant CG 0026

145   Participants CG 0021/0022

146   Participant CG 0006

147   Participant CG 0020

148 Participant CG 0013
149 Participant CG 0020
150 Ibid.
151 Ibid.
152 Participant CG 0006
153 Participant CG 0004
154 Participant CG 0013
155 Participants CG 0021/0022
156 Participant CG 0013
157 Ibid.
158 Participant CG 0004
159 Participant CG 0016
160 Participant CG 0004
161 Participant CG 0020
162 See "Money Matters."
163 Participant CG 0002
164 Participant CG 0006
165 Participant CG 0004
166 Participant CG 0033
167 Ibid.
168 Ibid.
169 *Self-care* is the act of focusing upon one's self as a caregiver to avoid "caregiver burnout" where one becomes ill or otherwise incapable of continuing to take care of their family member. Examples of self-care that may stave off caregiver burnout may include using respite help to take a break from the caregiving responsibilities, joining a support group, using humor or exercise, talking to doctors or counselors, self-educating and turning to outside help, adult day care, or even placement when necessary. (Source: Truman, K., *The Dementia Caregiver's Little Book of Hope*, 2009/2016)
170 Participant CG 0033
171 Ibid.
172 Participant CG 0008
173 Participant CG 0033
174 Participant CG 0007
175 Participant CG 0033
176 Ibid.
177 Participant CG 0007
178 Ibid.
179 Participant CG 0033
180 Ibid.
181 Participant CG 0016
182 See "Family Affair."
183 Ibid.

184 See "Money Matters."

185 Participant CG 0027

186 See "Storm Warning."

187 Participant CG 0016

188 Abstract Provided

189 CFP Board's *Academic Research Colloquium for Financial Planning and Related Disciplines*, February 7–9, 2017, in Washington DC

190 Participant CG 0016

191 Ibid.

192 Participant CG 0015

193 Ibid.

194 Participant CG 0024

195 Ibid.

196 Ibid.

197 Ibid.

198 Participant CG 0027

199 *Wandering* and *Exiting*: Wandering is sometimes used as a description for when an individual simply becomes unaware of their surroundings to the degree that they get lost. Their confusion may keep them from finding their way back to a still known place such as their home, or even where they last were with their friend or family member in a store, at a park, or other pubic place. When Alzheimer's- or dementia-afflicted individuals become confused about where they are residing (be it at home, an assisted living facility, or a memory care unit), they may exhibit "exiting" behaviors. Their desire to exit their present place so they may find something more familiar, possibly seeking to return to someplace where they believe they belong. Sometimes these locales no longer exist except for in the mind of the demented individual— such as a former place of employment or even a childhood home. These behaviors are not combative, but emerge from their confusion. However, they can place them into very dangerous circumstances, so caregivers can become quite stressed over trying to keep them in a safe environment.

200 Electronic tracking devices worn by the potential wanderer may help local law enforcement to more quickly locate a lost individual, while acting as an ID band. These GPS-based devices are desirable, but if no such service exists within a caregiver's area—they should still wear an ID band, with ailment and family notification information. Local Alzheimer's support groups or law enforcement agencies may be able to provide specific details for what types of tracking and/or ID devices may be available in one's area.

201 Participant CG 0024

202 Ibid.

203 Participant CG 0015

204 See *Note* 199. Industry professional's example: "If they're a 'walky-talky' they can maneuver around a facility, it's not a big deal—most times we have

secured courtyards…but if somebody walked in…sometimes it'd be nothing for them to just scoot behind them and 'exit seek.' I know one incident… the individual got lost in a cornfield because the facility was close to a cornfield—but they did find him. They don't have any knowledge that they're not supposed to be out of this protective area, but they recognize a whole world out there and they just go—they'll go." (Participant IP 0029).

205   Participant CG 0003

206   Participant CG 0019

207   Participant CG 0003

208   Ibid.

209   Participant CG 0014

210   Participant CG 0017

211   Participant CG 0011

212   Participant CG 0014

213   Ibid.

214   Participant CG 0011

215   Ibid.

216   Participant CG 0011

217   Participant CG 0003

218   Ibid.

219   Ibid.

220   Participant CG 0014

221   Participant CG 0006

222   Participants CG 0021/0022

223   Ibid.

224   Participant IP 0032

225   Participants CG 0021/0022

226   Ibid.

227   Participant IP 0032

228   Participant CG 0002

229   Participants CG 0021/0022

230   Participant CG 0013

231   Participant CG 0009

232   Participants CG 0021/0022

233   Participant CG 0002

234   Participant CG 0033

235   Ibid.

236   Participant CG 0030

237   Ibid.

238   Participant CG 0008

239   Participant CG 0033

240   Participant CG 0007

241   Participant CG 0033

242   Ibid.

243   Within multiple participants' transcripts, the terms *medfib* or *medical fib* were used as face-saving slang for a "white lie" by caregivers to appease their ill family members.

244   Participant CG 0016

245   Ibid.

246   Participant CG 0010

247   Ibid.

248   Participant CG 0016

249   Participant CG 0010

250   Participant CG 0027

251   Participant CG 0010

252   Participant CG 0015

253   Ibid.

254   Participant CG 0027

255   Ibid.

256   Participant CG 0024

257   Participant CG 0027

258   Participant CG 0024

259   Participant CG 0027

260   Participant CG 0024

261   Participant CG 0010

262   Participant CG 0027

263   Participant CG 0024

264   Participant CG 0010

265   Ibid.

266   Participant CG 0027

267   Participant CG 0016

268   Participant CG 0015

269   Participant CG 0027

270   Ibid.

271   Participant CG 0014

272   Participant CG 0019

273   Participant CG 0003

274   Participant CG 0019

275   Ibid.

276   Ibid.

277   Ibid.

278   Participant CG 0026

279   Participant CG 0011

280   Participant CG 0019

281   Participant CG 0014

282   Participant CG 0026

283 Ibid.

284 Johnathan Graff-Radford, MD, of the Mayo Clinic, has noted that music appears to continue to be received by individuals with Alzheimer's (even those without communication abilities) because musical memories may be retained in an area of the brain undamaged by the disease. This allows the caregiver to use music therapy as a diversion mechanism to soothe or occupy their loved one. Dr. Graff-Radford listed music's ability to "relieve stress, reduce anxiety and depression" and "reduce agitation," while additionally doing the same for the caregivers. (Graff-Radford, J., *Music and Alzheimer's: Can It Help?*, September 29, 2015, www.mayoclinic.org)

285 Participant CG 0026

286 Participant CG 0019

287 Participant CG 0026

288 Participant CG 0019

289 Participant CG 0004

290 Ibid.

291 Participant CG 0006

292 Participant CG 0013

293 Ibid.

294 Ibid.

295 Ibid.

296 Ibid.

297 Ibid.

298 Ibid.

299 Participant CG 0009

300 Ibid.

301 Participant CG 0013

302 Participant CG 0006

303 Ibid.

304 Ibid.

305 Participant CG 0004

306 Participant CG 0002

307 Ibid.

308 Participant CG 0004

309 Participant CG 0013

310 Participant CG 0023

311 Participant CG 0033

312 Ibid.

313 Ibid.

314 Ibid.

315 Participant CG 0008

316 Participant CG 0033

317 Ibid.

318   Participant CG 0007

319   Participant CG 0033

320   Participant CG 0007

321   Ibid.

322   Ibid.

323   Ibid.

324   Ibid.

325   Ibid.

326   Participant CG 0033

327   Participant CG 0007

328   Ibid.

329   Participant CG 0023

330   "The SilverSneakers® fitness program is a health plan benefit for Medicare beneficiaries that provides older adults with fitness center membership, customized group exercise classes, and a supportive social environment that promotes socialization among participants." Hamar, B., Coberley, C. R., Pope, J. E., and Rula, E. Y. (2013). "Impact of a Senior Fitness Program on Measures of Physical and Emotional Health and Functioning." *Population Health Management, 16* (6), 364–372.

331   Participant CG 0016

332   Ibid.

333   Ibid.

334   Ibid.

335   Participant CG 0015

336   Ibid.

337   Participant CG 0016

338   Ibid.

339   Participant CG 0027

340   Participant CG 0024

341   Participant CG 0016

342   Ibid.

343   Ibid.

344   Ibid.

345   Participant CG 0015

346   Participant CG 0016

347   Ibid.

348   Participant CG 0015

349   A *safety net* refers to the caregiver's backup plans to provide oversight and continuance of care should they no longer be able to function in their caregiver role. Caregiver burnout, health challenges of their own, or even predeceasing their ill family member—all require prior planning for putting this safety net into position. Without doing so places the very person they are caring for into peril upon their own health failure or death. Properly imple-

menting a safety net will follow clear discussion with the next person(s) in line to be caregiver(s) and incorporate these contingent fiduciaries into the appropriate legal documents.

350   Participant CG 0023
351   Participant CG 0015
352   Participant CG 0027
353   Participant CG 0015
354   Participant CG 0024
355   Participant CG 0016
356   Participant CG 0024
357   Participant CG 0015
358   Ibid.
359   Participant CG 0026
360   Participant CG 0014
361   Ibid.
362   Ibid.
363   Participant CG 0019
364   Participant CG 0003
365   Ibid.
366   Participant CG 0014
367   Ibid.
368   Participant CG 0011
369   Ibid.
370   Ibid.
371   Ibid.
372   Participant CG 0003
373   Participant CG 0019
374   Ibid.
375   Ibid.
376   Ibid.
377   Participant CG 0006
378   Participant CG 0020
379   Participant CG 0013
380   Participant CG 0023
381   Participant CG 0004
382   Participant CG 0013
383   Ibid.
384   Participant CG 0020
385   Participant CG 0002
386   Ibid.
387   Ibid.
388   Participant CG 0004
389   Participants CG 0021/0022

[390]   Ibid.

[391]   Ibid.

[392]   Ibid.

[393]   Participant CG 0033

[394]   Participant CG 0008

[395]   Participant CG 0033

[396]   Participant CG 0008

[397]   Ibid.

[398]   A "Category 1" hurricane is a tropical storm with sustained winds of 74 to 95 miles per hour on the Saffir-Simpson Hurricane Wind Scale—which rates hurricanes from Category 1 to Category 5. The National Hurricane Center of the National Oceanic and Atmospheric Administration (NOAA) states a Category 1 hurricane as having "very dangerous winds—will produce some damage." Source: www.nhc.noaa.gov

[399]   Ibid.

[400]   Ibid.

[401]   Ibid.

[402]   Ibid.

[403]   Participant CG 0033

Rock 'n' Roll to Rocking Chairs

[404]   Alzheimer's Association's Facts and Figures, 2017

[405]   Anticipated 40 to 46 million Alzheimer's caregivers is an extrapolation of the incidence of Alzheimer's—from the current 5.5 million increasing to between 13.8 to 16 million by 2050 and the estimated number of current Alzheimer's related caregivers of 15.8 million. Alzheimer's Association's *Facts and Figures*, 2017

[406]   Alzheimer's Association's *Facts and Figures*, 2017, p. 23.

[407]   Tiller, *Rock 'n' Roll to Rocking Chairs: Cognitively Impaired Baby Boomers' Impact and Liability for the Financial Industry* (working paper), poster and abstract published, CFP Board Academic Research Colloquium, 2017

Figure 13

Rock n' Roll to Rocking Chairs: Cognitively Impaired Baby Boomers' Impact and Liability for the Financial Industry

Robert W. Tiller, CFP®, CFS, RFC®

Doctoral Candidate ('17) University of South Florida MUMA College of Business

CFP BOARD — CENTER FOR FINANCIAL PLANNING

PROBLEM SCALE

More than $10 Trillion will be owned by cognitively impaired individuals in the United States by 2050, creating significant challenges and costs for the financial industry to protect them from financial exploitation.

ABSTRACT

An estimated 16 million Americans will have Alzheimer's disease or another form of memory disorder by 2050 and will be unable to act for themselves in their financial decisions.

The financial services industry these US Baby Boomers will be depending upon in retirement includes large and small brokerage firms, banks, credit unions, mutual fund companies, insurance companies, retirement plan custodians, alternative investment companies and independent wealth advisors.

This entire industry is now tasked with implementing procedures and protections to enable respectfully empowering older investors while also averting elder financial exploitation (most often by family members).

Analysis includes longevity and generational wealth data for the Baby Boomers, the terms and characteristics for dementia and cognitive impairment, the impact of aging on financial reasoning, the privacy problems and costs in the industry's adhering to US Treasury Department's Financial Crimes Enforcement Network (FinCEN) "red flags" for detecting financial exploitation, and the liabilities for failing to identify loss of capacity or simplify communications for seniors with limited reasoning.

Key findings are that even if efforts to protect against Elder Vulnerabilities become a major focus of industry regulators, research indicates the population volume and longevity of the Baby Boomers will lead to an alarming number of Americans becoming victims of elder financial exploitations.

INDUSTRY ANALYSIS METHOD

Public data from the US Department of Census, the US Council on Aging and other elder organizations.

Personal interviews with the Alzheimer's Family Organization's Executive Director, and Board Certified Elder Attorneys.

Academic journals and industry articles were sought via Google Scholar from keywords along three areas of research to explain, assess and interpret the current and future overlaps which exist between them:

RESEARCH SEGMENTS

Cognitive Decline and Decision Making for Older Persons
- What constitutes mild or severe cognitive decline, dementia or impairment?
- How do aging and/or cognitive impairment affect decision making?

Baby Boomer's Wealth and Preparedness for Incapacitation
- How much wealth will these problems involve?
- How have retiring Americans addressed Long-term care concerns?

Elder Financial Exploitation and Vulnerabilities
- What elder vulnerabilities exist today?
- What agencies and laws exist to protect against elder financial abuse?

What Constitutes Mild or Severe Cognitive Decline, Dementia or Impairment?

How Do Aging and/or Cognitive Impairment Affect Decision Making?

How Much Wealth Will These Problems Involve?

Composition of Total Individual Net Worth: Pre-Baby Boomer Generation / Baby Boomer Generation

Decline of Defined Benefit Plans

How Have Retiring Americans Addressed Long-Term Care Concerns?

Long Term Care 2006 Funding Sources

What Elder Vulnerabilities Exist Today?

Kathleen Quinn

What Agencies and Laws Exist to Protect Against Elder Financial Abuse?

What Financial Industry Obligations and Regulations on Elder Financial Abuse Exist?

REFERENCES

FUTURE RESEARCH

My doctoral dissertation project will be a practice informed, research book on a phenomenological study of caregivers with a CFM from differing familial relationships—ahead of the anticipated wave of cognitively impaired Baby Boomers.

CONTACT

robert.tiller@mail.usf.edu

USF MUMA

2017 Academic Research Colloquium for Financial Planning and Related Disciplines

Figure 14

Industry Analysis Abstract

Rock n' Roll to Rocking Chairs: Cognitively Impaired Baby Boomers' Impact and Liability for the Financial Industry

Tagline

More than $10 Trillion will be owned by cognitively impaired individuals in the United States by 2050, creating significant challenges and costs for the financial industry to protect them from financial exploitation.

Keywords

Cognitive Impairment, Elder Vulnerabilities, Financial Capacity, Inappropriate Family Fiduciaries, Negligent Denial.

Executive Summary

An estimated 16 million Americans will have Alzheimer's disease or another form of memory disorder by 2050 and will be unable to act for themselves in their financial decisions. The financial services industry these US Baby Boomers will be depending upon in retirement includes large and small brokerage firms, banks, credit unions, mutual fund companies, insurance companies, retirement plan custodians, alternative investment companies and independent wealth advisors. This entire industry is now tasked with implementing procedures and protections to enable respectfully empowering older investors while also averting elder financial exploitation (most often by family members).

Analysis includes longevity and generational wealth data for the Baby Boomers, the terms and characteristics for dementia and cognitive impairment, the impact of aging on financial reasoning, the privacy problems and costs in the industry's adhering to US Treasury Department's Financial Crimes Enforcement Network (FinCEN) "red flags" for detecting financial exploitation, and the liabilities for failing to identify loss of capacity or simplify communications for seniors with limited reasoning.

Key findings are that even if efforts to protect against Elder Vulnerabilities become a major focus of industry regulators, research indicates the population volume and longevity of the Baby Boomers will lead to an alarming number of Americans becoming victims of elder financial exploitations.

About the Author:

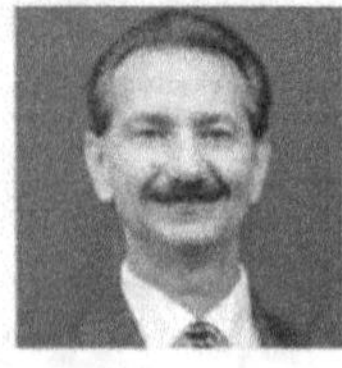

Robert W. Tiller, DBA ('17) is a doctoral candidate at the University of South Florida's Muma College of Business. He has been in the personal finance industry for over thirty years with individual practitioner and supervisory experience. His research focuses on the impact of America's aging for individuals, their families, the financial industry and the nation. He co-authored *21st Century Wealth: Essential Financial Planning Principles* in 2000 and was an invited guest for the *2015 White House's Conference on Aging.*

Figure 15

"Effective Net Worth" calculation explanation email excerpt:

February 2017:
(Fellow doctoral candidate's name removed),

Although the $10 trillion number seems staggering, the math is quite simple, (which is the scary part)—as my estimate surpassed that mark merely by multiplying the 16 million estimated afflicted individuals by their "Effective Net Worth" (ENW), i.e. total assets held in title _and_ their entitled incomes from pension and social security. (Note: The ballooning Social Security payment obligation to these individuals was not discounted for any future US Government reductions—which may or may not occur.)

My industry analysis paper cited multiple researchers, with differing aggregate net worth methods, whose estimates for Baby Boomers I was then able to include in my calculations—which yielded a per person range of $152,000 to $390,000 (without the ENW) and $680,000 to $847,000 with the ENW. Using the more conservative of the ENW amounts, $634,000 average ENW x 16 million estimated incapacitated by 2050 results in $10.88 trillion of financial resources that may belong to individuals lacking legal capacity. The non-ENW methods researchers' totals resulted in a range of $2.43 trillion to $6.24 trillion, whilst the highest ENW method estimated a potential $13.55 trillion. (I strongly believe ignoring the pension and Social Security resources is a significant error in researcher perspective—so, I stand firm by my ENW methodology instead.)

Please feel welcomed to cite my industry analysis working paper (as *Rock n' Roll to Rocking Chairs: Cognitively Impaired Baby Boomers' Impact and Liability for the Financial Industry* was publicly introduced via abstract and poster session at this month's Certified Financial Planner™ Board's Academic Research Colloquium in DC); or you could cite my forthcoming yet unnamed paper specifically theorizing *Effective Net Worth* (ENW) as a more accurate representation for an individual's financial measure (which was requested by FPA members at that ARC for me to more formally introduce it to the industry because neither compliance client profile forms nor financial planning software include such a measure yet).

I have included a partial reference list for you below, but I will spare you my preliminary notes on the ENW paper—which will most likely be a post-doc writing effort.

Have a great presentation at *(national financial firm's name removed)*.

Best regards,
Bob

Robert W. Tiller, CFP®, CFS, RFC®
DBA ('17) Candidate, University of South Florida

References:

2015 Alzheimer's disease Facts and Figures, Alzheimer's Association

The Disappearing Defined Benefit Pension and Its Potential Impact on the Retirement Incomes of Baby Boomers, B.A. Butica, et al, Social Security Bulletin, Vol. 69, No. 3, 2009

Are Baby Boomers Richer Than Their Parents? Intergenerational Patterns of Wealth Ownership in the United States, L.A. Keister, N. Deeb-Sosa, Journal of Marriage and Family, Vol. 63, Issue 2, 569-579, May 2001

The Wealth of the Baby Boom Cohorts after the Collapse of the Housing Bubble, D. Rosnick, D. Baker, Center for Economic and Policy Research, (2009)

Baby boomers and their parents: how does their economic well-being compare in middle age? Sabelhaus and Manchester, Journal of Human Resources, Vol. 30. No. 4, 1995, pp. 791-806

US Census Bureau, US Government Printing Office, Washington, DC, 2014

The retirement wealth of the baby boom generation, E.N. Wolff, Journal of Monetary Economics 54 (2007) 1-40

Considerations in the estimation of retirement wealth: Comments on "the retirement wealth of the baby boom generation: by Edward N. Wolff", A.B. Kennickell, Journal of Monetary Economics 54 (2007) 41-48

408 Issues may be studied at different levels and with differing research techniques best suited to attaining data from that particular level. Socioeconomic phenomena provides multiple perspectives, each of which may focus upon the same subject with different concerns, influencing factors and effects. Governmental action or reaction may be on a social issue also of interest to an individual citizen or family—yet their vantage, objectives, and concerns will be different. In case study research, once the unit of analysis has been identified, the kind of data to be collected and effective methods for obtaining such follows. *Forgotten Faces: Family Caregiver Voices* is based upon a research study that used the individual family level as the unit of analysis. However, this research perspective ahead of the wave of baby boomer cognitive impairment is intended to encourage further exploration of the subject at different units of analysis to broaden understanding. (Foundational source: Yin, *Case Study Research*, 2014)

409 Participant CG 0011

410 Participant CG 0023

411 *Stakeholder Theory*: Freeman's 1984 definition of stakeholders as "any group or individual who can affect or is affected by the achievement of the firm's objectives" (1984: 25) has been used in academic and business literature to describe the direct and indirect impacts of the actions (or absence of actions) by individuals, companies, governments, nature, or others. Whether the downline effects are taken into consideration (or not) may become the basis for adulation or criticism. Corporate responsibility and potential liability often draw upon stakeholder theory in framing opinions. This book has replaced the "firm's objectives" to that of an "ailment's ramifications," then used similar downline measures—to note the direct and indirect stakeholders of the phenomenon. This usage primarily differs from stakeholder theory, because firms' actions may be implemented by design, whereas Alzheimer's and dementia are merely occurring by happenstance. Akin to stating those affected by the ecological, financial, or psychological impacts of natural disasters would be considered stakeholders in such a happenstance incident.

412 Participant CG 0002

413 Mace and Rabins, *36-Hour Day*, 1981 John Hopkins University Press, 1999 revised.

414 The Alzheimer's Association's mission statement: "To eliminate Alzheimer's disease through the advancement of research; to provide and enhance care and support for all affected; and to reduce the risk of dementia through the promotion of brain health." (Alzheimer's Association website: alz.org, September 2017)

415 Medical journals and industry journals are the outlets for much of the scientific and academic research papers to be published. Those within the specific journals' fields may then draw upon that information for their own work. White papers are often shorter papers, outside of these industry journal arti-

cles, written to draw attention to an issue or development and are frequently published in business periodicals or posted to company websites. The public audience is generally informed by books, magazines, newspapers, television, radio, or other online venues (including websites), which draw from the information of the original research papers.

416   Obioha, A., *Noninvasive Eye Scan Could Detect Key Signs of Alzheimer's Disease Years Before Patients Show Symptoms*, CEDARS-SINAI, August 17, 2017 (source: https://www.cedars-sinai.edu/About-Us/News/News-Releases-2017/Noninvasive-Eye-Scan-Could-Detect-Key-Signs-of-Alzheimers-Disease-Years-Before-Patients-Show-Symptoms.aspx)

417   As an alternative for diagnosing Alzheimer's by measuring mental decline or by postmortem biopsy of brain tissue, biological markers or "biomarkers" are being sought to provide an earlier detection of the disease. Just as measuring "blood glucose" levels as a biomarker for diabetes, many fluids are being studied to locate a reliable indicator of Alzheimer's and/or other dementia ailments. Some of the biomarkers being considered will involve examining extracted cells from blood and other samples, while many are detected and analyzed by brain scan imaging. (Source: www.alz.org/research/science/earlier_alzheimers_diagnosis.asp#Biomarkers)

418   Byrne, Rodriques, Blennow, et al., "Neurofilament Light Protein in Blood as a Potential Biomarker of Neurodegeneration in Huntington's Disease: A Retrospective Cohort Analysis," *The Lancet Neurology*, June 7, 2017.

419   Participant CG 0011

420   Beckwith, Bill, *Managing Your Memory, Practical Solutions for Forgetting*, 2004/2010.

421   Mace and Rabins, *36-Hour Day*, 1981 John Hopkins University Press, 1999 revised.

422   Truman, Karen, *The Dementia Caregiver's Little Book of Hope*, Dementia Caregiver Resources Inc., 2016 revised.

423   Participant CG 0016

424   Katz, S. (1983). "Assessing Self-Maintenance: Activities of Daily Living, Mobility, and Instrumental Activities of Daily Living." *Journal of the American Geriatrics Society*, 31: 721–727.

425   Joshua M. Wiener, Raymond J. Hanley, Robert Clark, Joan F. Van Nostrand, "Measuring the Activities of Daily Living: Comparisons Across National Surveys," *Journal of Gerontology*, Volume 45, Issue 6, November 1, 1990, pp. S229–S237.

426   Participant CG 0016

427   Participant CG 0003

428   Participant CG 0027

429   Ibid.

430   Ibid.

431   Ibid.

432   Participant CG 0006

433   Participant CG 0009

434   Checkovich, Stern, "Shared Caregiving Responsibilities of Adult Siblings with Elderly Parents," *The Journal of Human Resources*, XXXVII, 3.

435   AARP, Caregiving in the US, 2015

436   Alzheimer's Association, *Facts and Figures 2015*, p. 31

437   Participant CG 0003

438   Participant CG 0004

439   Participant CG 0033

440   Participant CG 0007

441   Ibid.

442   Participant CG 0004

443   Ibid.

444   Participant CG 0026

445   A *fiduciary* is "an individual in whom another has placed the utmost trust and confidence to manage and protect property or money. The relationship wherein one person has an obligation to act for another's benefit." Source: fiduciary duty. (n.d.) *West's Encyclopedia of American Law, edition 2.* (2008). Retrieved September 13, 2017, from https://legal-dictionary.thefreedictionary.com/fiduciary+duty.

446   Health Insurance Portability and Accountability Act (HIPAA), effective in 2003, was developed by the US Department of Human Health and Services and was "designed to provide privacy standards to protect patients' medical records and other health information provided to health plans, doctors, hospitals and other health care providers." (Source: https://www.medicinenet.com/script/main/art.asp?articlekey=31785)

447   Participant CG 0004

448   Participant CG 0033

449   Participant CG 0004

450   Participant CG 0006

451   Tiller, Robert W., *Rock 'n' Roll to Rocking Chairs: Cognitively Impaired Baby Boomers' Impact and Liability for the Financial Industry*, abstract/poster published, CFP Board Academic Colloquium, February 2017.

452   Advisory to Financial Institutions on Filing Suspicious Activity Reports Regarding Elder Financial Exploitation, Department of the Treasury, FinCEN, February 2011.

453   Participant CG 0008

454   Corbin, K., "Who are the Perpetrators of Elder Financial Abuse?," *Journal of Financial Planning*, May 2015.

455   Ibid.

456   Participant CG 0004

457   Participant CG 0007

458 On May 24, 2018, the Senior Safe Act (SSA) became federal law. It provides immunity to financial institutions (and eligible individuals within them) "from liability in a civil or administrative proceeding for reporting potential exploitation of a senior citizen." While no action is mandated by the SSA, it details the training programs necessary to qualify for the stated immunities. Senior Safe Act Fact Sheet, FINRA, https://www.finra.org/sites/default/files/2019-05/senior_safe_act_factsheet.pdf

459 Tiller, Robert W., *Failure to Avert an Inappropriate Family Fiduciary*, FPA's Theory in Practice Circle webcast, March 2017.

460 Ibid.

461 Participant CG 0024

Money Matters

462 Kayne, Stephen H., Harrington, Charlene, LaPlante, Mitchell. (2010). "Long-Term Care: Who Gets It, Who Provides It, Who Pays, And How Much?" *Health Affairs*, 29, No. 1, 11–21.

463 Ibid.

464 Participant CG 0014

465 Tiller, Robert W., (working paper) *Medicaid Millionaires: The Ethics of Evasion*, 2017, submitted abstract:

ROBERT W. TILLER

Figure 16

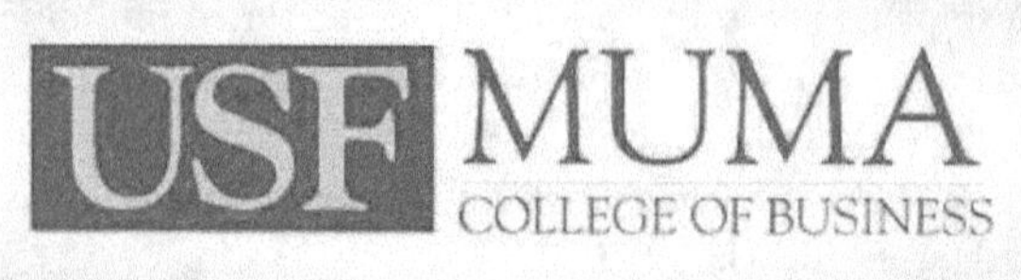

04/03/2016

Novel Idea Paper Cover Page

Medicaid Millionaires:
The Ethics of Evasion

Tagline

The impending wave of more than 72 million Baby Boomers becoming Elder Americans should expand the academic and professional dialogue surrounding Medicaid beyond historical review, costs of care or qualifying methodology to foster an open public discussion on the ethical perspectives involved. The trillions of dollars in anticipated Long-Term Care (LTC) costs this aging cohort will require leaves little doubt that sustaining the Medicaid Trust for the Baby Boomers and beyond will require significant funding increases or alterations for benefit qualification. At the heart of this financial and ethical discussion is the question, "Who should pay for Elder Americans' LTC?"

Keywords

Medicaid planning, Baby Boomers, Ethics, Fiduciary, Elderly Financial Exploitation

Executive Summary

Each day millions of US tax dollars are spent by Medicaid as a safety-net for the nation's impoverished elderly population's LTC expenses—yet Medicaid recipients have often "qualified" for benefits by transferring away substantial assets instead of spending them down on their own care. Before the Baby Boomers' LTC needs "Bust the Medicaid Trust," an exploration on the ethics in avoiding Medicaid's spend-down provisions is warranted. This paper will briefly explain the history of Medicaid, examples of qualifying standards and common techniques for circumventing spend-down rules, the US government's challenges for enforcing the "Granny Goes to Jail Act" or the "Granny's Lawyer Goes to Jail Act," and demonstrate that the answer of who should (or should not) be entitled to use Medicaid Trust funds differs by perspective. Are Medicaid benefits solely for the poor? How much should individuals be entitled to keep of what they worked a lifetime to save? Is it ethical for advisers to direct families on how to shelter wealth instead of spending it down? Why does the Federal Government cover health problems such as Cancer, Diabetes or Joint Replacements for elders as a part of Medicare, but leave the States and individuals to pay for Alzheimer's disease and other LTC ailments? What would constitute an elderly person's "fair share" of their LTC costs? Does that "fair share" differ between the Middle-Class or Millionaires? The various ethical interpretations behind the emotional perspectives will be examined against the financial backdrop of America's impending Medicaid crisis.

466   Ibid.

467   Participant CG 0011

468   Ibid.

469   Participant CG 0014

470   R. J. Carney, et al. 2002. "Can We Still Fund Long-Term Care Financing Without Buying a Policy, and Do We Want To?" *Managerial Finance*, Vol. 28, Issue 7, pp. 9–26.

471   Sharp, Cynthia. 2015. "What Every Lawyer Needs to Know about Planning for Retirement," *GP Solo*, Vol. 32, Issue 6, 42–45.

472   Tiller, Robert W. 2015. *Alzheimer's Family Organization*. Working discussion case.

473   Takacs, Timothy, McGuffey, David. 2002. "Medicaid Planning: Can It Be Justified? Legal and Ethical Implications of Medicaid Planning." *Wm. Mitchell Law Review*, 111–158.

474   Tiller, Robert W. 2016. *Rock 'n' Roll to Rocking Chairs: Cognitively Impaired Baby Boomers' Impact and Liability for the Financial Industry*. Abstract/poster published. CFP Board Academic Colloquium, February 2017.

475   Participant CG 0015

476   Tiller, Robert W., (working paper) *Medicaid Millionaires: The Ethics of Evasion*, 2017.

477   Sharp, Cynthia. 2015. "What Every Lawyer Needs to Know about Planning for Retirement." *GP Solo*, Vol. 32, Issue 6, 42–45.

478   Karp, Joseph, Gershbein, Sara. 2005. "Poor on Paper: An Overview of the Ethics and Morality of Medicaid Planning." *The Florida Bar Journal*. October 2005, 61–65.

479   Driscoll, Marilee. 2004. "Medicaid Planning Primer for Financial Advisers." *Journal of Financial Service Professionals*. January, 65–74.

480   Participant CG 0019

481   Participant CG 0026

482   The Veterans Administration provides some benefits for veterans (or a single surviving spouse of a veteran) who served at least 90 days, part of which must have been during wartime—may (not *will*) be eligible for the VA's Aid and Attendance program.

Qualifying information may be obtained through links to the Pension Management Center for each state or the VA Facility Locator directly on the VA's website: https://www.benefits.va.gov/pension/aid_attendance_house-bound.asp

The Aid and Attendance (A&A) increased monthly pension amount may be added to your monthly pension amount if you meet <u>one</u> of the following conditions:
- You require the aid of another person in order to perform personal functions required in everyday living, such as bathing, feeding, dressing,

attending to the wants of nature, adjusting prosthetic devices, or protecting yourself from the hazards of your daily environment
- You are bedridden, in that your disability or disabilities requires that you remain in bed apart from any prescribed course of convalescence or treatment
- You are a patient in a nursing home due to mental or physical incapacity
- Your eyesight is limited to a corrected 5/200 visual acuity or less in both eyes; or concentric contraction of the visual field to 5 degrees or less

(Source: www.va.gov)

It bears repeating that transfers of assets out of an individual's name to qualify for Aid and Attendance may be counted as a part of the five-year lookback for Medicaid qualification—or disqualification. Individuals or families considering VA A&A benefits would be wise to seek appropriately credentialed professionals, well versed in both VA and Medicaid benefits.

[483] Ibid.

[484] Participant CG 0014

[485] Alzheimer's Association's *Facts and Figures*, 2017, p. 18

[486] Participant CG 0026

[487] Tiller, Esperiti, Peterson, et al., *21st Century Wealth: Essential Financial Planning Principles*, 2000.

[488] Financial Services Institute's Forum *The Changing Face of Retirement*, coinciding with the 2012 Republican National Convention in Tampa, Florida.

[489] Tiller, Robert W., 2016, *Rock 'n' Roll to Rocking Chairs: Cognitively Impaired Baby Boomers' Impact and Liability for the Financial Industry*, abstract/poster published, CFP Board Academic Colloquium, February 2017.

[490] Retirement calculators are available from most financial planners, many investment or insurance professionals, and online with most banks, insurance companies, or financial services firms. When discussing, with their financial professionals, the various investment mechanisms most appropriate for providing them a lifetime income, differences or similarities to their parents' health, longevity, and risk level should factor into the amount necessary to equal or surpass their parents' pensions.

[491] Re: Effective Net Worth (ENW)
In the past 20 years, nearly every client, compliance officer, software provider, and several financial advisors I've mentioned ENW to have agreed with the logic and wondered why it hasn't become mainstream. A state senator at the 2012 *The Changing Face of Retirement* forum was disappointed when I told him my private financial services firm used the calculation in-house, but it wasn't part of the industry's compliance methods for determining "liquid" or "investable" net worth.

At the 2017 CFP Board's Academic Colloquium, I reintroduced ENW by mentioning it in one of my poster presentations. An attendee who taught finance suggested it be more formally incorporated into a paper and submitted to an economics or finance journal to potentially have it become better known. I thanked him for his interest and told him I would do so sometime after I completed the book on the caregiver study I was doing. While it would be satisfying to see other scholars accept the concept, it is more important to find a means for introducing it more broadly into practice.

It is primarily the public who does not understand the importance of building an adequate ENW—as banks and brokerage firms do give some consideration to these income streams for loans or investment suitability, yet without plainly communicating such back to the consumer. While industry and government may be able to help improve the public's financial knowledge, neither is responsible for doing so. I would encourage both to advance the public's financial acumen, as the alternative could be grave for the state Medicaid programs' solvency.

Behind the Curtain

[492]   Metro-Goldwyn-Mayer Inc., 1939, *The Wizard of Oz*, film based on Baum, L. F., & Granger, P. (1958). *The Wizard of Oz*. New York: Scholastic Book Services.

[493]   See *Note* 9.

[494]   See *Note* 2.

[495]   Human Subjects Research is subject to the guidelines set forth by the National Institute of Health (NIH) with certification of educational courses on Human Subjects Research required to move forward on "research involving a living individual about whom an investigator obtains either data through interaction or identifiable, private information." This book's research study was subject to the approval of an Institutional Review Board, as mandated by the NIH requirements.

⁴⁹⁶ Figure 17

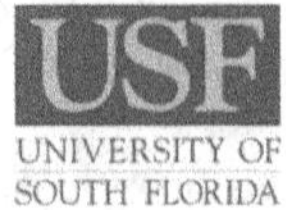
UNIVERSITY OF
SOUTH FLORIDA

Informed Consent to Participate in Research
Information to Consider Before Taking Part in this Research Study
IRB Study # 00030013

We are asking you to take part in a confidential research study called **"Caregiver to a Cognitively Impaired Family Member Phenomenon."** The purpose of this study is to learn about individuals' experiences when caring for a cognitively impaired family member.

This study involves one 45-90 minute in-person interview with a researcher.

The person in charge of this research study is Robert Tiller, a doctoral candidate and the Principal Investigator. However, other research staff may be involved and can act on behalf of the person in charge. He is being guided in this research by his dissertation co-chairs: Dr. Anand Kumar and Dr. Richard Will.

The research will be conducted in person.

Purpose of the study

The purpose of this study is to:

- Explore individuals' experiences when caring for a cognitively impaired family member at differing familial relationship levels, (spouse to spouse, child to parent, etc.), to provide an in-depth insight and understanding of the issues, concerns, challenges and events future caregivers in a similar role may experience.

Study Procedures

We are asking you to take part in this research study because you are/were a primary or secondary caregiver, directly or indirectly responsible for the Activities of Daily Living and well-being of a cognitively impaired relative.

If you take part in this study:

Participants will be individually asked to describe their caregiver to a cognitively impaired family member experiences in a private and confidential in-person interview with the Principal Investigator, Robert Tiller.

Local primary and secondary caregiver participants are welcomed to be interviewed together, and individual participants are welcomed to have a non-participating family member or friend sit with you during the interview, if desired.

The first part of the interview format will consist of participants' answering background and pre-impairment information to familiarize the Principal Investigator with the study participants and to properly categorize their relationship with their cognitively impaired family member.

Figure 18

Participants will then be asked open-ended questions for them to share their own accounts of what they experienced as in their caregiver role.

As the participants explain their caregiver experiences, the Principal Investigator may ask for clarification or situational examples to assure accuracy of their perspective.

Throughout the interview, participants are welcomed to ask for clarification of any questions or comments made by the Principal Investigator, and may request a pause—then decide to continue, reconvene at another time, or simply end the session.

At the conclusion of the interview, all caregiver participants will be given the contact information of a local caregiver support group they may call for emotional support or professional guidance.

Participants will also be welcomed to call Robert Tiller the week following their in-person interview, to avoid them feeling they had missed an opportunity to relate some additional information they believe important to communicate about their caregiver experience.

The entire study interview should take between 45-90 minutes for the participant.

Interviews will be recorded for transcription. These recordings will be kept confidential. Identifying information of the interviewees will be kept in a password protected file accessible to only the researcher.

Total Number of Participants

Approximately 50 individuals will take part in this study at USF

Benefits

The potential benefits of participating in this research study may include: imparting wisdom to benefit future caregivers, validate and enhance purpose of participant's family's circumstances, and a cathartic release by sharing own story with a confidential, concerned audience.

Risks or Discomfort

This research is considered to be minimal risk. That means that the risks associated with this study are the same as what you face every day. There are no known additional risks to those who take part in this study.

Compensation

Participants will not be compensated.

Privacy and Confidentiality

We will keep your study records private and confidential. Certain people may need to see your study records. By law, anyone who looks at your records must keep them completely confidential. The only people who will be allowed to see these records are:

- The research team, including the Principal Investigator, Advising Professors, his dissertation committee and all other research staff.

- Certain government and university people who need to know more about the study. For example, individuals who provide oversight on this study may need to look at your records. This is done to make sure that we are doing the study in the right way. They also need to make sure that we are protecting your rights and your safety.

215

Figure 19

- The USF Institutional Review Board (IRB) and its related staff who have oversight responsibilities for this study, staff in the USF Office of Research and Innovation, USF Division of Research Integrity and Compliance, and other USF offices who oversee this research.

We may publish what we learn from this study. If we do, we will not include your name. We will not publish anything that would let people know who you are.

Alternatives / Voluntary Participation / Withdrawal

You do not have to take part in this study. You should only take part in this study if you want to volunteer. You should not feel that there is any pressure to take part in the study. You are free to participate in this research or withdraw at any time.

You can get the answers to your questions, concerns, or complaints

If you have any questions, concerns or complaints about this study, or experience an adverse event or unanticipated problem, email Robert Tiller at roberttiller@XXXX.XXX.XXX.

If you have questions about your rights as a participant in this study, general questions, or have complaints, concerns or issues you want to discuss with someone outside the research, call the USF IRB at (813) 974-5638.

Consent to Take Part in Research

It is up to you to decide whether you want to take part in this study. If you want to take part, please read the statements below and sign the form if the statements are true.I freely give my consent to take part in this study.I understand that by signing this form I am agreeing to take part in research. I have received a copy of this form to take with me.

____   ___________________

Signature of Person Taking Part in Study   Date

____

Printed Name of Person Taking Part in Study

Statement of Person Obtaining Informed Consent

I have carefully explained to the person taking part in the study what he or she can expect from their participation. I confirm that this research subject speaks the language that was used to explain this research and is receiving an informed consent form in their primary language.This research subjecthas providedlegally effective informed consent.

____   ___________________

Signature of Person Obtaining Informed Consent   Date

____

Printed Name of Person Obtaining Informed Consent

Version #2 05/22/17   Page 3 of 3

497   Participant CG 0009
498   Ibid.
499   Participant CG 0016
500   Participant CG 0019
501   Participant CG 0016
502   Participant CG 0014
503   Ibid.
504   Participant CG 0016
505   Participant CG 0008
506   Participant CG 0007
507   Participant CG 0007
508   *Time to Share*, music and lyrics by Cameron Washburn, performed by *PKRB*

Research Reflections

509   *Conceptual schemes* are "models" used to "think" about phenomena without presenting theories. Rather, they are research models to build understanding, placing "usefulness" ahead of absolute truths—which may be "communicated effectively" but "recognizes its own limitations." T. Grandon Gill, (2011), "When What is Useful is Not Necessarily True: The Underappreciated Conceptual Scheme," *Informing Science: The International Journal of an Emerging Trans-discipline*, Vol. 14.
510   Participant CG 0016
511   Participant CG 0030
512   Participant CG 0020
513   Participant CG 0023
514   Participant CG 0014
515   Participants CG 0021/0022
516   Ibid.
517   Participant CG 0013
518   Participant CG 0020
519   Participant CG 0033
520   Participant CG 0024
521   Participant CG 0020
522   Participants CG 0021/0022
523   Ibid.
524   Participant CG 0007
525   Participant CG 0014
526   Participant CG 0003
527   Participant CG 0014
528   Participant CG 0003
529   Participant CG 0007
530   Ibid.
531   Participant CG 0014

About the Author

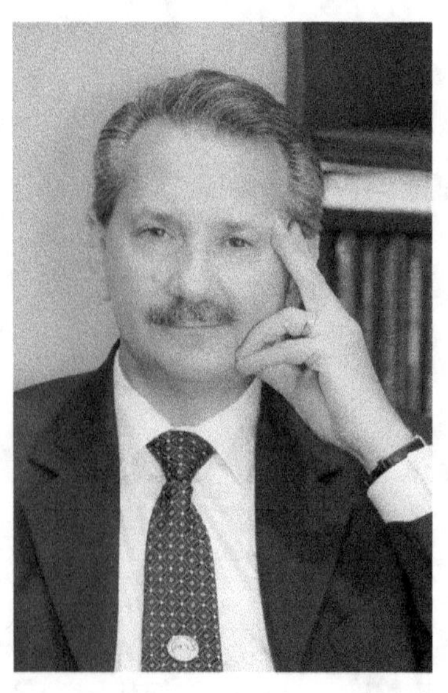

Robert W. Tiller, D.B.A., CFP®, RFC® is a practitioner-scholar who, after more than three decades of private practice in personal finance, became an independent researcher, an Adjunct Professor, and then the Director of the Personal Financial Planning degree program at the University of South Florida. He earned his Doctorate of Business Administration to complement his Certified Financial Planner™ Professional and Registered Financial Consultant designations acquired previously.

Dr. Tiller was a contributing author for *21st Century Wealth: Essential Financial Planning Principles* in 2000, a primary panelist for the Financial Services Institute's 2012 *The Changing Face of Retirement* forum and an invited focus group participant at the 2015 *White House Conference on Aging*. His research focuses upon the impact of aging for elderly investors, their families, and the challenges faced by future retirees.